Perioperative Practice
Fundamentals of Homeostasis

John Clancy, Andrew J. McVicar and Nicola Baird

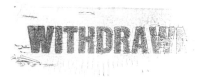

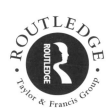

LONDON AND NEW YORK

First published 2002
by Routledge
11 New Fetter Lane, London EC4P 4EE

Simultaneously published in the USA and Canada
by Routledge
29 West 35th Street, New York, NY 10001

Routledge is an imprint of the Taylor & Francis Group

Typeset in Sabon by Wearset Ltd, Boldon, Tyne and Wear
Printed and bound by Gutenberg Press Ltd, Malta

British Library Cataloguing in Publication Data
A catalogue record for this book is available from the British Library

Library of Congress Cataloging in Publication Data
Clancy, John.
    Perioperative practice : fundamentals of homeostasis John Clancy, Andrew J. McVicar,
and Nicola Baird.
        p. cm.
    Includes bibliographical references and index.
        1. Operating room nursing. 2. Surgical nursing. 3. Homeostasis. I. McVicar, Andrew J.
II. Baird, Nicola, 1962– III. Title.
RD32.3 .C56 2002
610.73'67—dc21
                                                                              2001048953

        ISBN 0-415-23310-0 (hbk)
        ISBN 0-415-23311-9 (pbk)

Contents

Figures

Colour plates

Tables

Boxes

Foreword

The human body is a complex and fascinating organism. Put it in water and it can prevent itself from becoming waterlogged, overload it with salt and it will rapidly react by re-establishing the correct degree of salinity. Deplete it of blood, and it will bring into play forces which will ensure that the brain, heart, lungs, kidneys and other essential organs receive the best of a diminishing blood supply. How it does all of these things is still not entirely understood. However, the concept of homeostasis allows us to study this incredibly complex environment and apply some sort of understanding to the variety of systems which make up the human body.

Why is the concept of homeostasis important to perioperative practitioners?

This is a crucial question because, in my opinion, the concept of homeostasis underpins the core objectives of perioperative practice and as such directs and guides the activities which constitute that practice.

So, indulge me for a minute. As you read this foreword, let your imagination take over and imagine that you are a practitioner, supporting your patient as he undergoes a complex surgical procedure.

The patient is lying in the ward waiting for a member of the surgical team to come and take him to theatre. He has already suffered a huge assault on his body – the accident that he was in has shattered his leg. As he lies there, his body is vainly trying to restore some sort of normality to his system. The broken leg resulted in almost a fifth of his total blood volume being lost to the circulation. The result was that blood pressure and pulse were affected, which in turn led to the blood flow to vital organs being compromised. Fat emboli released from bone marrow into his blood threaten to damage the circulation and the biochemical composition of his blood is causing serious imbalances leading to potential kidney and lung problems. If the patient survives this initial assault on his system, the bone would eventually heal, but only with major loss of function. The body simply cannot cope with the extent of the trauma. The sensitive and delicate balance between the body systems has failed and urgent action must be taken.

When homeostasis is compromised in this way, the medical interventions that take place are aimed at restoring the balance in order for the body's own healing processes to come into play. In this preoperative phase of the patient's care, fluid will be replaced, electrolytes will be assessed and balanced, blood will be transfused, the broken bone will be immobilised and the pain will be controlled. All these measures will help to prevent further injury and will temporarily support the body systems during the crucial early stages following the injury. However, it is not enough. Unless the injury is repaired, the patient will be, at best, severely compromised, and at worst may even die. Surgery is required.

The second major assault on the patient's body is about to begin. In order to gain access to the damaged site, skin must be cut, breaking the natural barrier to infection and the outside environment. Muscle fibres are split or cut and bone is stripped of its periosteum, manipulated, reduced and fixated. Sensory receptors identify these activities and responses and act to bring the body's systems back within their normal range of function. Unaided, these will inevitably fail and the system will quickly succumb to chaos as the systems swing wildly out of control.

This then is the aim of the multidisciplinary perioperative team: to support and reinstate the normal homeostatic mechanisms of the body while the damage to the broken bone is repaired. This support will include administering fluids and electrolytes to replace those lost during surgery; preventing infection and encouraging the normal repair of damaged tissues; maintaining blood flow to the vital organs; ensuring a steady supply of oxygen to the tissues; and eliminating pain and anxiety and their associated physiological effects. All this and more is the objective of medical interventions during this patient's surgery.

Perioperative practitioners, as part of the multidisciplinary team, play their part in administering and monitoring the effects of these interventions and as such, play a vital part in restoring the body to a healthy state. The core objective of a practitioner's role is therefore to promote homeostasis through either reinforcing adaptive physiological responses, or providing extrinsic support to make those responses more effective, or reducing the impact of responses that are maladaptive and therefore detrimental. This practice is humanised by developing a holistic approach to the care and support of the patient as a whole; a concept which fits comfortably within a broader interpretation of homeostasis.

It was this understanding of the vital function that practitioners play in the support of the body systems that led Kate Nightingale, a previous editor of the *British Journal of Perioperative Nursing*, to commission John Clancy and Andrew McVicar to write a series of articles on homeostasis which form the basis of this book. These were then succeeded by a further series looking at the anatomical and physiological changes brought about by surgery.

I believe that an understanding of anatomy and physiology is essential to underpin perioperative practice, and as such I have been happy to support and encourage the publication of this core text. I am sure that you, the perioperative practitioner, will find this insight into the body's systems equally as fascinating.

Paul Wicker BSc, RMN, RGN, CCNS (Operating Department Nursing), PG Cert in Teaching and Learning. Programme Leader, Operating Department Practice Education, Edge Hill College of Higher Education, Liverpool; Editor, *British Journal of Perioperative Nursing*.

About this book

This book examines some important physiological principles applied to perioperative practice.

The opening chapter introduces the reader to the anatomical construction of the human body, emphasizing the planes of the body, common terms of relative position and examines the content of the body cavities – all basic but essential information necessary for the 'newcomer' to the perioperative environment. The chapter also explores in depth the principles of homeostasis from a health–illness perspective.

Why *homeostasis*? The concept of homeostasis typically is one of a constant performance or environment, but in physiology such an interpretation is not strictly correct because there must be scope for adaptation to allow people to achieve developmental milestones, or to change performance level according to need. Homeostasis in the physiological sense therefore represents a dynamism that is central to human functioning. Nevertheless, the concept remains about control; few processes in the body occur by chance, and those that do promote corrective or adaptive responses. This book is especially concerned with identifying the adaptive responses to the trauma of surgery. The intention is to utilize homeostasis as a framework to aid learning and so help students and perioperative practitioners appreciate the physiological basis of practice.

Chapter 2 explores the surgical approach from two perspectives. First, it considers issues related to gaining access to tissues and organs in 'open' surgery, and second, it considers the uses of endoscopes in 'minimal access surgery'. Gaining access to deep tissues entails crossing the skin, skeletal muscle and associated blood vessels and nerves, and this chapter would not be complete without attention being drawn to the relevant anatomy and physiology of these structures.

The third chapter considers body fluid homeostasis. The homeostatic roles of electrolytes in body fluid compartments are explained, and the possible impact of surgery on body fluid volume and composition are identified. The physiological principles underpinning common infusates are also discussed.

Chapter 4 introduces the reader to the fundamentals of immunity. This understanding is essential: patients entering hospital may already have an infection, may acquire one whilst in hospital awaiting for operation, and are susceptible to infection during and after the surgical procedures. This chapter also details the homeostatic responses associated with the wound healing process.

The fifth chapter explores the essential anatomy and physiology of the cardiovascular system and common related pathophysiological conditions and important diagnostic indicators. The principles of shock and its prevention during the perioperative period and an overview of pharmacology associated with re-establishing cardiovascular homeostasis are also considered.

Perioperative influences on respiratory homeostasis are discussed in Chapter 6. The chapter identifies the importance of cellular respiration, the distinction between respiratory acidosis and alkalosis, and the principles of blood gas homeostasis. Perioperative influences on pulmonary function are highlighted, and ventilation therapy as a homeostatic mechanism is explored.

In Chapter 7 the associated physiological responses of stress that may arise during surgery are considered. Surgical stress is discussed on three fronts: stress related anxiety, the stress relationship with general anaesthesia and stress responses to trauma.

The final chapter details the neurophysiology associated with the 'gate' control theory to explain the subjective nature of perception pain. The gate theory is also utilized in explaining the physico-biochemical rationale of perioperative pain relief.

Whilst the book assumes some knowledge of physiology, it identifies and explains the main aspects of function that in turn relate to homeostatic disturbance arising through surgical procedures. Application Boxes are used throughout to reinforce how perioperative care acts to minimize or reverse functional disturbance, and its consequences.

Reader exercises and reflective questions are included within the text and illustrations of each chapter to test the reader's understanding. Some questions will require further reading to enhance the reader's understanding of physiological processes; in such instances the reader is directed to, in particular, Clancy, J. and McVicar, A.J. (2002). *Physiology and Anatomy. A Homeostatic Approach. Second Edition*. London: Arnold.

Although each chapter can be read individually, the reader is strongly encouraged to first read Chapter One since the principles discussed and, in particular, the inclusion of a simple but unique feature, the homeostatic graph, are the foundations for what follows in the other chapters. Indeed frequent cross-referencing with other chapters is used to highlight where the processes described integrate with those of other systems.

Finally, we hope you enjoy reading the book, and that it contributes to a better understanding of perioperative care between the practitioner and the patient, to the ultimate benefit of both.

Happy reading   John Clancy, Andrew McVicar, Nicola Baird
2002

P.S. We would welcome comments on the value of this book so that the next edition will evolve!

Acknowledgements

The time from the conception to production of *Perioperative Practice: Fundamentals of Homeostasis* has been long and we would like to take the opportunity to thank the people who have helped and encouraged us along the way.

In particular our special thanks go to:

Paul Wicker, the Editor of the *British Journal of Perioperative Nursing* who commissioned two series of articles comprising over twenty papers, which lay the foundations of this book. His enthusiasm for the concept was a driving force.

Others whose contributions to those articles made us rethink some of the content of the book:

Louise Dye, formerly a Theatre Staff Nurse, Bupa Hospital, Norwich; Anne-Marie Ramsay, Staff Nurse, Norfolk and Norwich University NHS Trust; Mriga Williams, Senior Lecturer, Anglia Polytechnic University and Janet Cox, Clinical Practitioner, In-patients Theatres, Norfolk and Norwich University NHS Trust. Their expertise in theatres has made the homeostatic graph come alive in aspects of perioperative nursing care. Louise, Janet and Ann-Marie are former students who have (hopefully!) been inspired by our teaching: Thanks go to you all.

Colleagues for their continued support, in particular Sophia Pike for emergency typing, Annette Wilson, Technical Secretary, for her assistance with the illustrations, Sue Sides, Penny Goacher, for putting up with our moans and groans when we were working to deadlines.

Our employers, the University of East Anglia and Anglia Polytechnic University, Norfolk and Norwich University NHS Trust, for their support and help with resources.

The reviewers, whose excellent reviews and evaluative feedback provided the motivation to produce this book.

The Editorial and Production Teams at Routledge for their advice, support, enthusiasm, skill and investment in the text. Edwina for the nice lunches – I hope they continue!

Finally a note to our families: Rachel, Penny and children Lauren, Clare and Lisa for their support.

Our very special parents Ann and Norman Clancy, James and Mary McVicar, Jim and June Baird.

John Clancy, Andrew McVicar, Nicola Baird
2002

Figure and table acknowledgements

The authors would like to thank the following for their kind permission to use illustrative material in this book.

Hodder Arnold

Figures 1.2, 1.6, 2.1a–b, 2.2, 2.3, 4.1, 4.3, 4.4, 4.5, 4.6, 4.8, 4.10, 4.11, 4.12, 5.2a-b, 5.5, 5.6, 8.1, 8.2, 8.3, 8.4, 8.5, 8.6a–b, 8.7, 8.8, 8.11, Plates 4i–vi and Tables 1.1, 4.1, 4.3, 4.4 originally published in Clancy, J. and McVicar, A. (2002) *Physiology and Anatomy: A Homeostatic Approach, 2nd edition*, London: Arnold.

British Journal of Theatre Nursing (now *British Journal of Perioperative Nursing*)

Figure 4.2 from Clancy, J. and McVicar, A.J. (1997) 'The essentials of immunology' 7(1):17–26.
Figure 4.9 from Clancy, J. and McVicar, A.J. (1997) 'Wound healing: a series of homeostatic responses' 7(4): 25–33.
Figure 5.7 adapted from McVicar, A.J. and Clancy, J. (1996) 'Hypoxia: a respiratory imbalance. A homeostatic imbalance' 6(10): 15–20.
Figures 5.8, 5.9 and 5.10 from McVicar, A.J. and Clancy, J. (1996) 'Shock: a failure to maintain cardiovascular homeostasis' 6(6): 19–25.
Figures 4.5 and 4.6 from McVicar, A.J. and Clancy, J. (1997) 'Influence of surgery on body fluid homeostasis' 7(8): 27–32.
Figure 7.6 from McVicar, A.J. and Clancy, J. (1998) 'The metabolic response to surgery' 8(3): 12–18

Table 1.2 from Clancy, J. and McVicar, A.J. (1996) 'Homeostasis: the key concept in physiological studies' 6(2): 17–24.
Tables 4.2, 4.3 and 4.6 adapted from Clancy, J. and McVicar, A.J. (1997) 'Wound healing: a series of homeostatic responses' 7(4): 25–33.
Table 4.5 from Clancy, J. and McVicar, A.J. (1997) 'Wound healing: a series of homeostatic responses' 7(4): 25–33.
Table 8.1 from Clancy, J. and McVicar, A.J. (1998) 'Perioperative pain management: a gate control perspective' 7(14): 15–24.

Chapter 1

The human body and principles of homeostasis

Introduction

This book is about anatomy and physiology; the two branches of science that will help you understand the human body. Identifiable within these sciences is the central concept referred to as homeostasis.

Definitions

- Human anatomy refers to the study of the structure of the body.
- Physiology is concerned with the mechanisms of human bodily function.
- Homeostasis refers to the automatic, self-regulating processes necessary to maintain the 'normal' state of the body's environment despite changes in the environment outside the body.

Collectively, anatomical structure, physiological function and the maintenance of homeostasis enable the body to attain the basic needs necessary for health and a 'normal' life. Before contemplating the principles of homeostasis, the reader should become familiar with how the body is organized.

Anatomical organization

The outside of the human body has a definite and recognizable shape; the inside contains the organs, which are specifically located relative to each other. The anatomical position of the body provides a reference point when studying or describing the position of body structures. This position is when the person stands erect, facing forward, with arms at his/her side with palms facing forwards. For example, organs such as the heart are drawn according to this convention, so those features on the left side appear on the right, almost as though the observer is looking into someone's chest.

> ## Box 1.1   Application: positioning the patient on the operating table
>
> The position of the patient on the operating table usually depends on the operation being carried out and the surgeon's preference. The needs of the anaesthetist are also considered, since the position must enable him/her to maintain anaesthesia in complete safety. However, the patient may have a predisposing condition, which prevents the preferred position from being used and an alternative or revised position must be sought. It is important for the perioperative practitioner to have an in-depth knowledge of the various table positions (Figure 1.1 p. 4) and the equipment required for each case. Particular attention is applied to patient safety; the operating table is very narrow and the patient must be placed securely on the table. The use of pressure relieving devices is essential as patients can remain in one position for several hours, and ischaemic changes to areas exposed to pressure can cause pressure areas/sores, potentially prolonging the patient's hospital stay. Over-extension of joints and limbs must be avoided; poor positioning can lead to nerve and muscle damage and dislocation of joints. Any exposed areas of the body, which may come into contact with metal (table or attachments), must be protected to avoid inadvertent diathermy burns. Some positions might have special requirements, making them complex and time consuming to achieve, possibly involving a number of personnel.

A set of standard anatomical terms is used to describe each part of the body, the position of body structures and their geographical relationships with each other. Many of these regional terms are illustrated in Figure 1.2. The main terms used relate to 'planes of the body', 'relative positioning of organs' and 'body cavity' (see below, p. 5).

Planes of the body

Body structures are described by the perioperative practitioner in relation to three planes or imaginary lines which run through the body. These are called median (or mid-sagittal), transverse (or horizontal) and coronal (or frontal) lines (Figure 1.3). The median plane passes directly along the mid-line of the body, dividing the body into perfectly symmetrical right and left halves. The transverse plane passes horizontally through the body dividing it into upper and lower portions. The coronal plane divides the body into front and back portions.

Terms of relative position

The perioperative practitioner needs to understand the position of structures relative to each other and also to use directional terms (see Figure 1.3). For example: anterior and ventral are used interchangeably and refer to the front surface of the body. They also have a broader meaning, in the sense of a structure being closer

EXERCISES

1 Review the common surgical procedures employed when the patient is placed in the positions identified in Figure 1.1a–f and identify the equipment required for each surgical procedure cited.

2 Match the pressure areas indicated by Lists A, B and C – with the following positions
   a The supine position is associated with the pressure areas identified in List ____
   b The lateral position is associated with the pressure areas identified in List ____
   c The prone position is associated with the pressure areas identified in List ____

List A	List B	List C
Medial and lateral	Toes	Calcaneus
Malleolus	Patella	Sacrum and coccyx
Greater trochanter	Male genitalia	Thoracic vertebrae
Ilium	Breast	Scapulae
Ribs	Acromion process	Occiput
Ear	Cheek	
Acromion process	Ear	

See the end of this chapter for the answers to question 2.

to the front of the body. As an example: 'anterior abdominal wall' or 'the heart is anterior to the spine'. In the same way, posterior may refer to the back surface of the body or it may mean a structure is nearer to the back of the body. For example, the oesophagus (food pipe) is posterior to the heart. 'Dorsal' is similarly linked to 'posterior'. Likewise medial indicates that a structure is towards the mid-line of the body, whereas lateral designates that a structure is away from the mid-line of the body. 'Proximal' indicates that the structure concerned is nearer the attached end of a limb or thus the trunk of the body, whilst a 'distal' structure is farther away from the attached end of a limb and the trunk. For example, the humerus is proximal to the radius, whereas the phalanges are distal to the carpals.

EXERCISES

Look up in a biological dictionary what the following terms mean: afferent, efferent, peripheral, deep, superficial, internal and external.

Identify the location of the following bones: humerus, radius, phalanges and carpals.

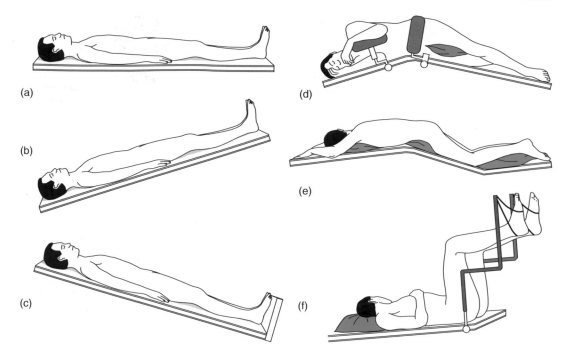

(a)

(b)

(c)

(d)

(e)

(f)

Figure 1.1 **Common positioning of the patient for various surgical procedures:**
a   the supine position,
b   the Trendelenburg position,
c   the reverse Trendelenburg position,
d   the lateral position,
e   the prone position,
f   the lithotomy position.

Perioperative practitioners must be familiar with the terminology used in theatre, speaking the same language, to avoid mistakes. Early in the practitioner's career, the anatomical terminology may be unfamiliar and difficult to understand. But once the practitioner has mastered an understanding of basic words, including prefixes (the beginning of a word), roots (the main body of the word) and suffixes (the ends of words) you will be able to apply these principles to derive the meaning of terminology. For example, once you understand the prefix: 'electro-', means electrical, the root 'cardiac' refers to the heart and the suffix '-gram' means recording, then the meaning of the term 'electrocardiogram' becomes apparent.

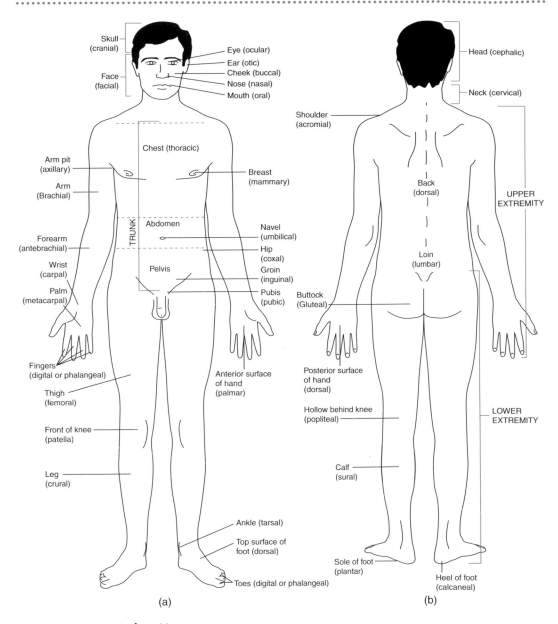

Figure 1.2 **Anatomical position**

The common names and anatomical terms (indicated in brackets) for many of the regions of the human body.

a   anterior view,

b   posterior view.

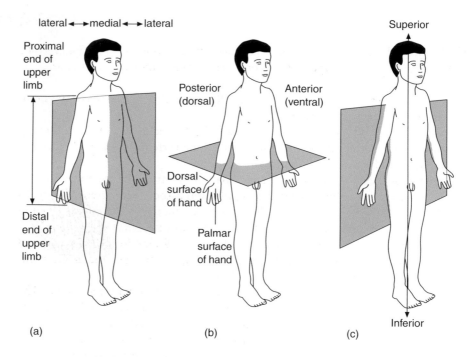

lateral ←→ medial ←→ lateral

Proximal
end of
upper
limb

Distal
end of
upper
limb

Posterior
(dorsal)

Anterior
(ventral)

Dorsal
surface
of hand

Palmar
surface
of hand

Superior

Inferior

(a)   (b)   (c)

Figure 1.3 **Planes through the body:**
a   medial (midsagittal) plane,
b   transverse plane,
c   coronal (frontal) plane.

Q. Which plane divides the body into:
a   anterior and posterior parts?
b   right and left parts which are mirror images of each other?
c   superior and inferior portions?

Q. Is the hip proximal or distal to the knee?

Body cavities

The body can be divided into cavities produced by the bony skeleton (Figure 1.4), and these contain the internal organs (or viscera). The main body cavities are:

■ the cranial cavity. The bones of the skull enclose this. This cavity accommodates and protects the brain.
■ the spinal cavity. This is formed by a hole (foramen = 'window') running through the vertebral column. This is called the vertebral canal and it accommodates and protects the spinal cord.
■ the thoracic cavity. This is the upper cavity of the trunk of the body. Its confines are the breastbone (or sternum), ribs and associated intercostal muscles (inter- = between, -cost = rib) and cartilage, vertebral column, diaphragm and the structures below the neck. The cavity contains the windpipe (or trachea), two lungs, the heart and its great vessels, the food pipe (or oesophagus) and associated nerves and lymphatic supply. The space between the lungs, occupied by the heart, is called the mediastinum.
■ the abdominal cavity. This is the large lower portion of the trunk. The diaphragm, the pelvic cavity, the spine, abdominal muscles and lower ribs confine it. It accommodates the organs concerned with digestion and absorption of nutrients, and other organs associated with these functions. These are the gall bladder, liver, spleen and pancreas. In addition the kidneys, ureters (superior regions) and adrenal glands are also located in this region.
■ the pelvic cavity. This is the lowest portion of the trunk, a continuation of the abdominal cavity. Its boundaries are the bony pelvis, sacrum and muscles of the pelvic floor. In the female it contains all the reproductive structures; in the male, however, only some reproductive structures are contained. The cavity of both sexes contains the ureters (lower regions), bladder and urethra. Other pelvic organs are part of the small intestine and the last part of the colon, the rectum and anal canal. It also includes the openings for the urethra, vagina (in the female) and anus.

Blood vessels, lymphatic nodes and associated nerves are located in all the cavities.

Sometimes it is necessary to be more precise in locating organs within the body. Thus the body is further subdivided into quadrants and the nine regions associated with the abdomen and pelvic areas (see Figure 1.5). This level of precision is required to determine the sites for surgical incision.

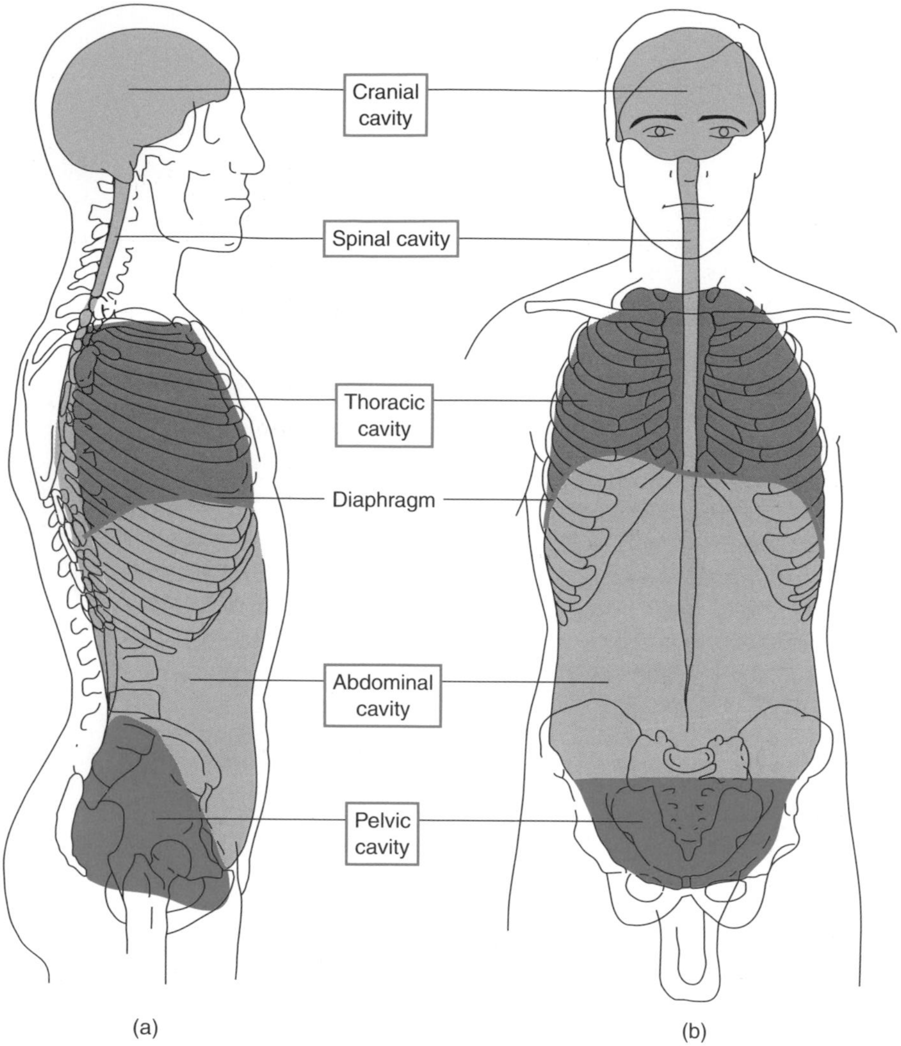

Figure 1.4 Lateral and anterior views of the human body showing major cavities:
a right lateral view,
b anterior view.

Q. What are the confines of the following cavities:
 i thoracic cavity,
 ii abdominal cavity,
iii pelvic cavity.

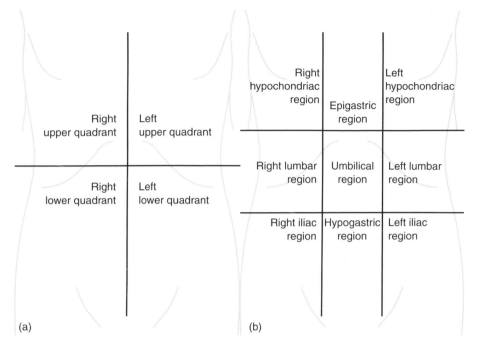

Figure 1.5 **Anatomical sub-divisions of the abdomen and pelvic regions:**
a   quadrants of the abdomen,
b   the nine regions of the abdominal and pelvic regions.

Q. Identify the quadrant that confines the stomach.

Q. Which region confines the appendix?

Box 1.2   Application: surface anatomical landmarks

Surface anatomy is the study of external structures and their relation to deeper structures. For example, the breastbone (sternum) and parts of the ribs can be seen and felt (palpated) on the anterior aspects of the chest. These structures can be used as landmarks to identify regions of the heart and points on the chest at which certain heart sounds can be heard using a stethoscope (a process called auscultation). The normal 'lub-dup' sounds of the heart reflect normal structure and functioning of the heart valves (see Figure 5.3). A change in sounds, to the trained ear, possibly reflects abnormal structure and/or functioning.

Anatomical imaging involves the use of x-rays, ultrasound, computerized tomographic (CT) scans and other technologies to create pictures of internal structures. Both surface anatomy and anatomical imaging provide important information in diagnosing disease. The perioperative practitioners swill become familiar with such techniques during their training.

EXERCISES

1 Using appropriate terminology describe the anatomical location of the organs of the thoracic and pelvic cavities of the body in relation to the 'border margins' of the named cavity.

2 Look up the prefixes associated with each major organ within the five major cavities of the body.

3 Match up the sites of incision in List 1 with the most likely operations in List 2

List 1
A right iliac fossa
B mid line
C loin above iliac crest
D suprapubic

List 2
1 prostatectomy
2 nephrectomy
3 appendectomy
4 partial gastrectomy
5 left lower lobectomy

A	B	C	D

Note: The suffix -ectomy means removal of, or cutting out, therefore appendectomy means the removal of the appendix.

4 Describe what is meant by the clinical term 'colectomy'.

5 Using a nursing or medical dictionary look up the following common prefixes and suffixes: per-, gastr-, mast-, -sonic, hemi-, -otomy, -scopy, -tome, trans-.

6 Match up the operation in List 1 with its description in List 2

List 1
A cholecystectomy
B cholangiogram
C choledocholithotomy
D choledochostomy

List 2
1 Opening common bile duct and draining
2 Removal of stones from the bile ducts
3 Removal of the gall bladder
4 A radiological film of hepatic, cystic and bile ducts after insertion of radiopaque dye.

A	B	C	D

See the end of this chapter for the answers to questions 3 and 6.

The basic needs of the human body and activities of daily living

The basic needs of the living body identified by biologists as the characteristics of life are:

1 feeding or nutrition. This encompasses the intake of raw materials to maintain life processes such as growth, repair and the maintenance of a normal environment inside the body.
2 movement. This is a characteristic in that people, or some part of them, are capable of changing their position.
3 respiration. This refers to the processes concerned with the production of the energy necessary to maintain life processes and movement. In humans it involves breathing (external respiration) and the breakdown of food (internal respiration) inside the cells of the body.
4 excretion. This is the removal from the body of waste products of chemical reactions, and of excesses of certain dietary substances (for example water).
5 sensitivity and responsiveness. These are the processes concerned with monitoring, detecting and responding to changes in the environment inside and outside the human body.
6 growth. This generally implies an increase in size and complexity. It also includes repair of body parts, which have undergone damage or need to be replaced.
7 reproduction. This is necessary for the continuation of the species.

Henderson (1996) reported that to help nurses direct care to the basic needs of the body, Roper *et al.* in 1990 devised a nursing model called the Activities of Daily Living (ADL). These are:

■ breathing,
■ eating and drinking,
■ elimination,
■ mobilizing,
■ controlling body temperature,
■ maintaining a safe environment,
■ sleeping,
■ personal cleaning and dressing,
■ working and playing,
■ communication,
■ expressing sexuality,
■ dying.

Surgical intervention may be necessary if one or more of these ADL were to be compromised to a degree that affects the quality of human life.

It must be understood that human beings are complex organisms having cellular, tissue, organ and organ system levels of organization (Figure 1.6).

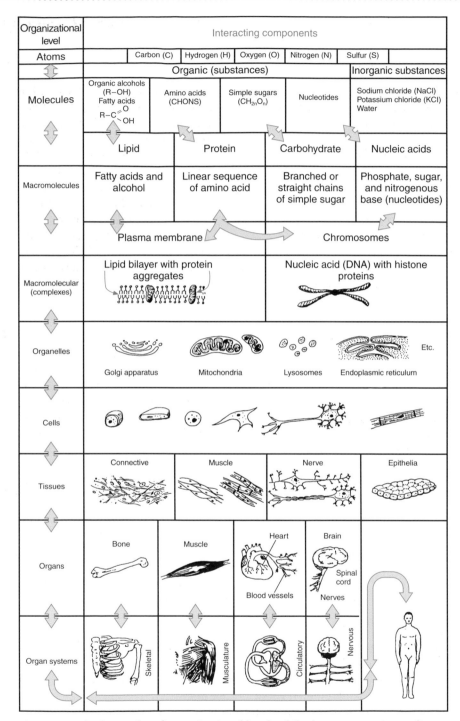

Figure 1.6 **The hierarchy of organizational levels of the human organism indicates that specific interactions at each simpler level produce the more complex level above it**

Levels of organization

Cellular

The human body is composed of trillions of microscopic cells. Each cell is regarded as a 'basic unit of life', since it is the smallest component capable of performing most, if not all, of the basic activities. Cells can digest food, generate energy, move, respond to stimuli, grow, excrete and reproduce. For example, mitochondria perform cellular respiration, lysosomes digest materials that have entered the cell. To facilitate cellular function throughout the body, the body contains many distinct kinds of cells, each specialized to perform specific functions. Examples include blood cells, muscle cells and bone cells. Each has a unique structure related to its function. Genes are the controllers of cellular function and these act indirectly through their role in enzyme production. Enzymes therefore are of fundamental importance in the human body since they control the speed of chemical reactions so that they are compatible with a healthy life. Hence genes are commonly referred to as the 'code of life' and enzymes the 'key chemicals of life'.

Tissue

A tissue is defined as a collection of similar cells and their component parts, which perform specialized functions. There are many different types of tissues and so it follows that there must be different cell types that comprise these tissues, bearing in mind the definition. However, the entire body consists of just four primary tissues: epithelia or lining tissues, binding or connective tissues, muscular tissues and nervous tissues.

Organ and organ system

An organ is an orderly grouping of tissues, which provide it with discrete function. Examples of organs are the heart, spleen, ovary and skin. Most organs contain all four primary tissues. In the stomach, for example, the epithelial lining performs functions of secretion of gastric juice and absorption of some chemicals such as alcohol. The wall of the stomach, however, also contains muscle tissue (for contraction of the stomach) to help with the breakdown of food, nervous tissue (for regulation) and connective tissue, which binds the other tissues together.

An organ system is a group of organs that act together to perform a specific body function, for example the respiratory system maintains the level of oxygen and carbon dioxide in the blood. These systems work with each other in a co-ordinated way to maintain the functions of the body.

Each level of organization is instrumental in sustaining the functions of life for the human body. Table 1.1 illustrates each organ system's involvement in the regulation of the basic needs of the individual.

Table 1.1 Organ system involvement in maintaining the basic needs of the human body

Basic needs		Organ systems involved
Intake of raw material	Food	Digestive
	Oxygen	Respiratory
Internal transportation		Circulatory and lymphatic
Excretion		Urinary, respiratory and the skin
Sensitivity and irritability	Environment outside the body	Special senses, nervous, skeletomuscular
	Environment inside the body	Nervous and endocrine
Defence	External (outside the body)	Skin and special senses
	Internal (inside the body)	Immune, digestive and endocrine
Movement within the environment		Skeletal, muscular, nervous and special senses
Reproduction		Reproductive and endocrine

NB: The Table demonstrates that all the organ systems are involved in maintaining the normal environment needed by the cells of the body, to enable them to perform the basic needs of the individual's health.

Box 1.3   Application: illness – a cellular imbalance!

Ultimately, every illness originates from a disturbance arising at a cellular level. In summary, this can be because of:

■ an environmentally induced expression of a gene which produces an excess of enzyme and the product of the metabolic reaction controlled by the enzyme, predisposing the individual to an illness; or
■ an environmentally induced repression of a gene that leads to insufficient enzyme concentration, hence reduction in the product of the metabolic reaction controlled by the enzyme, predisposing the individual to an illness; or
■ the gene may be absent resulting in an absence of a chemical, inducing a deficiency disease or syndrome.

The interdependence of the components of the body means that a failure of one function leads to a deterioration of others. This is reflected in the diverse signs and symptoms of ill-health that require clinical intervention to restore health (or homeostasis). For example, a patient who has had a myocardial infarction (heart attack) may display signs and symptoms that reflect poor functioning of the heart, lungs and kidneys.

The basic needs are interdependent. For example, we must take in the raw materials of food and oxygen in order to provide sufficient energy to maintain normal body function. This energy is needed to support chemical reactions, such as those involved in growth and in the muscle contraction necessary for movement. Consequently, these raw materials can be viewed as being the 'chemicals of life'. Chemical reactions also produce waste products; these wastes must be removed from the body to prevent cellular disturbances.

The interdependence of the basic needs means that a failure of one function leads to a deterioration of others. For example, malnutrition (mal- = bad, or poor) results in the retardation of growth and development, lethargy, poor tissue maintenance, a reduced capacity to avoid infection and a general failure to thrive.

In the context of this introductory chapter it therefore seems logical first to establish the basis for optimum (ideal) biological functioning. The main topic reviewed in the remainder of this chapter is therefore homeostasis.

Homeostasis: the link with health and ill-health

An introduction to homeostatic control theory

The word 'homeostasis' translates as 'same standing' and is usually taken to indicate constancy or balance. Those students who have entered healthcare in recent years having studied courses that have had a significant human biology component are likely to have come across the term, since it is an important concept, especially in physiological studies.

The idea that a constancy of the internal environment of the human body is essential to life can be traced to the views of the eminent French physiologist Claude Bernard, in the mid-nineteenth century. The turn of the twentieth century produced many important discoveries involving hormonal and neural regulation of the body.

In order to perform the basic functions of life successfully there must be a 'consistency' within the body, and in particular of the environment inside cells, called the intracellular fluid (intra- = inside). The regulation of the composition and volume of fluids that surround cells, which collectively are called the extracellular fluids, maintains environmental consistency. The main components of these fluids are detailed in Chapter 3 and are as follows:

1 tissue fluid. This is the fluid in which body cells are bathed. It acts as an intermediary between the cells and blood.
2 plasma, the cell-free component of blood. This fluid together with blood cells circulates through the heart and blood vessels, supplying nutritive materials to cells and removing waste products from them.

Two processes by which the composition of these fluids is kept constant are:

■   the intake of raw materials,

■ the removal (excretion) of waste products of chemical reactions, or of excesses of chemicals that cannot be stored, destroyed or transferred to other substances inside the body.

Conventionally, homeostasis is considered to represent a balance or equilibrium between these two processes.

Box 1.4   Application: perioperative multidisciplinary team – external agents of homeostatic control!

Homeostasis represents the processes necessary for the maintenance of conditions under which cells, and hence the body, can function optimally. For example, even small changes in body temperature, pH, or hydration can disrupt biochemical activities within a cell and may even kill it. The disruptions to homeostasis, if not carefully monitored and controlled by the anaesthetist and surgeon (assisted by the perioperative practitioner) could in the extreme be lethal for the patient intraoperatively, or delay recovery post-operatively and hence prolong the date of discharge from hospital. In summary, perioperative care is aimed at redressing (where possible) homeostasis for the patient/client. Health promotion and health education is directed at sustaining homeostasis for individuals within a population. Thus the multidisciplinary team could be considered external agents of homeostatic control.

The modern view is that homeostasis is dependent upon an integration of physiological functions, since all the organs of the body perform functions that help to maintain these constant conditions.

Organ systems therefore are homeostatic controllers that regulate the environment within cells throughout the body (Figure 1.7). This book concentrates on the homeostatic principles of human physiology, emphasizing the role of the cardiovascular and respiratory systems in the maintenance of an optimal cellular environment. The reader is actively encouraged to look at other texts for a detailed account of how organ systems interact to maintain cellular homeostasis.

Homeostasis is usually considered to pertain to physiological or biochemical processes and, for the bulk of this text, we will apply these principles. However, we also intend, where appropriate, to discuss homeostasis pertaining to psychophysiological consistency within the body. Not separating the mind ('psychological') from bodily ('physiological') functions is important because the cells making up the human brain are no different in their basic characteristics from any other cells in the body. This is significant when considering the metabolic stress response to surgery and pain. Thinking, emotions, behaviour and memories are all subjected to the same physical and chemical laws of other functions of the body. Thus to understand health fully it is therefore necessary to be familiar with the psychophysiological processes that account for individual differences, as well as with the principles of homeostasis. In summary, individual differences are

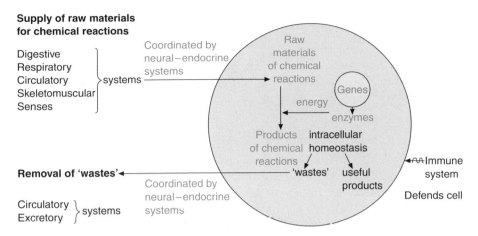

Figure 1.7 Organ system's involvement in regulation of intracellular homeostasis

Q. Suggest why the following statements are used in physiology:
a genes – 'the code of life',
b enzymes – 'the key chemicals of life'.

determined by a person's genes (i.e. nature), which are modified by environmental factors (i.e. nurture). The person and their environment are therefore inseparable. Thus, it is necessary that the nature–nurture implications of a person's health, ill-health and the need for surgery should be recognized, as these interactions provide the foundations of healthcare in general.

Principles of homeostasis

Cannon introduced the actual term 'homeostasis' in 1932 and defined it as: 'A condition, which may vary, but remains relatively constant.'

It was this definition, plus experience gained working alongside nurses and midwives using clinical laboratory values (see Table 1.2, Box 1.5), that inspired two authors of this book (Clancy and McVicar) to design the homeostatic graph (Figure 1.8). This simplified model aids the understanding of the association of a patient's physiological and biochemical parameters in health and disease.

The readers of this text are strongly recommended to familiarize themselves with this figure before 'dipping' into other chapters, since variants of it are used throughout this book as a model to explain:

1 homeostatic principles,
2 how components of homeostatic control function,
3 how failure of components of control results in illness,
4 an individualized approach to care, in which perioperative interventions are used to re-establish homeostasis for the patient.

The homeostatic range

The variations in parameter values provide a range within which the parameter can be considered to be regulated. The fluctuation in parameter values within their normal (homeostatic) range provides the optimal condition in the body (see Table 1.2, Figure 1.8). The range reflects:

- *the precision by which a parameter is regulated.* Some parameters, such as body temperature, have a very narrow range, whilst others, for example blood volume, have a relatively larger homeostatic range.
- *individual variation of values within the population.* One person's normal range could fluctuate just above the minimum values of the range (Figure 1.8, label a_1), whilst another person's optimal range could fluctuate close to the maximum values (Figure 1.8, label a_2). It is also considered normal for some individuals to deviate from either side of the mean (or average) value (Figure 1.8, label a_3). To account for all individual variations within the population, it is also possible for some individuals to 'bounce' between the minimum–mean–maximum values (Figure 1.8, label a_4).
- *variation of values within each person according to the changing metabolic demands.* It is quite usual for some parameters' maximum and minimum values to vary within the individual as one passes through the different developmental stages of the lifespan. The dotted lines associated with the maximum, mean and minimum values on Figure 1.8 indicate the dynamic nature of these values. That is, for some parameters, the maximum value may increase. For example, it is generally well known that blood pressure increases with the age of a population, whilst most other parameter values decrease with adult age (for example, muscle strength, visual acuity).

During illness and disease requiring surgery, variation can occur. Variations can also occur perioperatively because of the stress of surgery, which has an impact upon metabolic activity (see Chapter 7) and causes pain (see Chapter 8).

Normal variations exist which are associated with the individual's sleep–wake activities (or circadian patterns, circa- = about, -dies = day). Perioperatively any potential variation must be noted and accommodated; that is, appropriate interventions are employed to restore homeostasis.

The maintenance of a constant arterial blood pressure is frequently cited in textbooks as an illustration of a homeostatic process at work. However, it is important that this pressure is naturally increased during exercise as it increases blood flow through the exercising muscle ensuring that the oxygen supply to the muscle supports the increased demand. The elevation of blood pressure in exercise is itself a homeostatic adaptive process. It acts to provide the appropriate environment for the changing chemical needs of muscle, and this highlights the most important feature of homeostasis: physiological processes provide an optimal environment for bodily function. Whilst this may involve a near-constancy of some aspects of the environment (e.g. brain temperature), other functions may require a controlled change.

Table 1.2 Clinical chemistry laboratory values

Patient's surname	Patient's age/ date of birth
Patient's forenames	Hospital
Patient's consultant/GP	Ward
Date and time of specimen	

Clinical chemistry	Normal values (Homeostatic range)
Sodium	136–148 mmol/l
Potassium	3.8–5.0 mmol/l
Bicarbonate	24–32 mmol/l
Urea	2.6–6.5 mmol/l
Creatinine	60–120 umol/l
Glucose	Random 3.0–9.4 mmol/l
CSF glucose	2.5–5.6 mmol/l
Total protein	62–82 g/l
Albumin	36–52 g/l
Globulin	20–37 g/l
Calcium	2.2–2.6 mmol/l
Transaminase	up to 35 IU/l
PH	7.35–7.45
pCO_2	4.7–6.0 kPa
pO_2	11.3–14.0 kPa

Q. Describe in scientific terms what is meant by the term 'normal range' when equated with the values expressed in clinical laboratory tables.

Homeostasis, then, is about the provision of an internal environment that is optimal for cell function at any moment in time despite the level of activity of the individual. Health occurs when bodily function is able to provide the appropriate environment. This usually entails an integration of the functioning of physiological systems, the outcome is observed as physical well being and psychological equilibrium. In order for homeostasis to be maintained, the body must have a means of detecting deviations (or changes) to homeostasis, of assessing the magnitude of the deviation and of promoting an appropriate response to redress homeostasis (a process known as 'feedback'). Feedback processes also provide the means of assessing the effectiveness of the response

Receptors and control centres

The initial change in a physiological parameter is detected by sensory receptors, sometimes referred to as monitors or error detectors. The function of these receptors is to relay information about the disturbance to homeostatic control centres

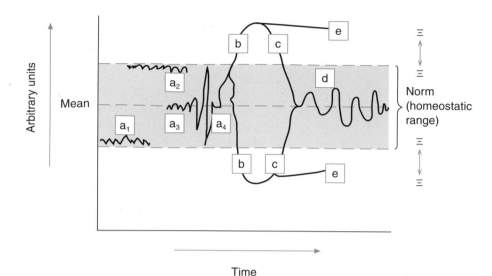

Time

Figure 1.8 **Principles of homeostatic control:**
a   1–4 homeostatic dynamism – values fluctuating within the homeostatic range –
    reflecting individual variation within the population with time of day and
    developmental stage of life (see text, p. 18, for details),
b   homeostatic imbalance,
c   homeostatic control mechanisms operating to restore homeostasis,
d   homeostasis re-established,
e   failure of homeostatic control mechanisms resulting in illness or death.

**Q. Suggest how the homeostatic range accounts for every individual in
the population**

(analysers or interpreters). These centres interpret the change as being above or
below the homeostatic range and determine the magnitude of the change. As a
result they stimulate appropriate responses via effectors that bring about the correction of the imbalance in order to restore homeostasis. Once the parameter has
been normalized the response will cease (see Figure 1.9a–b, p. 24).

Homeostatic controls

Occasionally, only one homeostatic control mechanism is necessary to redress the
balance. On occasions blood glucose concentration exceeds its homeostatic range
(a condition called hyperglycaemia, hyper- = over or above, glyc- = glucose, -emia
= blood). This results in the release of the hormone insulin, which promotes
glucose removal from blood. More frequently, a number of controls are involved.
For example, when the blood acidity exceeds its homeostatic range (a condition

> ## Box 1.5   Application: clinical normal and abnormal values
>
> In science 'normal' means conforming to the usual pattern. The normal (homeostatic) range in statistical terms defines values of parameters expected for 95 per cent of the population, for example, the normal range of blood pH is 7.35–7.45 (Table 1.2). Statistically, this means that 95 per cent (i.e. 95 out of 100 people) of the population have a pH within this range. Thus the homeostatic range of a parameter is useful in making judgements regarding the health status of an individual. However, it must be noted that each person is unique. Those 5 per cent of the population (i.e. 5 out of 100 people) whose pH is outside the 'normal' range are not necessarily abnormal or ill. These values reflect minor deviations from the homeostatic range and are considered to be 'acceptable' in clinical practice, and so need no clinical adjustments. Alternatively, values that reflect sudden and large deviations from the homeostatic range are considered 'unacceptable'. This is referred to as a homeostatic 'imbalance' or 'disturbance' and one in which perioperative intervention may not only be desirable, but essential to sustain 'normality' for the patient.
>
> Reference is made to clinical blood chemistry measurement perioperatively to ensure that no extreme deviation occurs. Not all patients have biochemical screening pre-operatively; fit healthy patients may only have their vital signs monitored. Patients with other medical problems will be screened accordingly; for example, diabetic patients will have their blood glucose levels estimated and measured. Patients 'booked for' or 'due to undergo' major surgery will require more extensive investigations.

referred to as an acidosis) three controls attempt to return the acidity values to the normal range. These are:

- buffers. These chemicals act to neutralize the excess acidity (see Chapter 3).
- respiratory mechanisms. If the buffers are insufficient in resolving the acidosis then the rate and depth of breathing will increase in order to excrete more carbon dioxide, a potential source of acid in body fluids (see Chapter 6).
- urinary mechanisms. If the increased rate and depth of breathing are insufficient to resolve the acidosis, then the kidneys will produce a more acidic urine, thus reducing the acidity of body fluids.

These corrective responses are time dependent; some are rapid responses to the imbalance, but if they should fail to re-establish homeostasis, other control mechanisms are prompted to correct the disturbance. The body therefore has short-term, intermediate and long-term homeostatic control mechanisms (Figure 1.9c). In the above example, these are the buffers, respiratory and urinary mechanisms respectively.

Homeostatic feedback mechanisms

Negative feedback

Most homeostatic control mechanisms operate on the principle of negative feedback. That is, when a homeostatic imbalance occurs, then in-built and self-adjusting mechanisms come into effect that reverse the disturbance. The regulation of blood glucose demonstrates the principle of negative feedback control. An increase in blood glucose concentration above its homeostatic range sets into motion processes that reduce blood glucose. Conversely, a blood glucose concentration below its homeostatic range (hypoglycaemia) promotes processes that will increase the blood glucose. In both situations, the result is that the level of blood sugar is kept relatively constant over periods of time.

> **EXERCISE**
>
> Using the information in this chapter, the reader should be able to identify the in-built, self-adjusting homeostatic mechanisms that are responsible for reversing elevated blood glucose concentration and acidity.

Positive feedback

However, there are times when actually promoting a change, rather than negating it, is of benefit. This is known as positive feedback. An example is observed in blood coagulation. When there is damage to the skin and its blood vessels, initiation of a positive feedback is a necessary mechanism in an attempt to stop blood flow (a process called haemostasis, see Chapter 4).

Homeostasis and ill-health

If homeostasis provides a basis for health, then ill-health will arise when there is a failure of the components of the control processes involved (Figure 1.9c–d). Imprecise control mechanisms include:

- receptors that fail to respond adequately to changes in the environment, and/or
- homeostatic control centres that fail to analyse sensory information, and/or analyse the information incorrectly and/or send incorrect information to the effector organs, and/or
- effector organs that fail to respond to corrective directions from the control centres.

Failure to provide an optimal internal environment will cause further destabilization. Thus an induced change in the activities of one part of the body may have far-reaching consequences for whole body function.

Disorders requiring surgical intervention are characterized by a primary disturbance of intracellular homeostasis within tissues somewhere in the body. Disease may be classed according to this primary disorder, for example a respiratory problem, a degenerative disorder, a tumour of a particular tissue, or due to immune system dysfunction or infection. However, all will have consequences for extracellular homeostasis, and hence the functioning of cells and tissues other than those involved in the primary disturbance. Thus perioperative care may be directed at symptoms apparently removed from the primary problem, for example relieving constipation in a patient with a breast tumour.

Box 1.6   Application: homeostasis and the nursing process

Homeostatic principles are readily discerned within the stages of the nursing process (compare Figure 1.9b and 1.9d). For example:

1 *assessment and nursing diagnosis.* The assessment of the health deficit, perioperative needs of the individual patient and the biological, psychological, social and spiritual needs of the individual correspond to the detection and assessment of change by the receptors of the homeostatic control mechanism.

2 *planning.* The planning of perioperative nursing care, based on the assessment (and in some specialities, diagnosis stage), is comparable to the ways by which homeostatic controls analyse and determine the responses needed to correct the imbalance. Furthermore, just as the body has specific homeostatic controls for different parameters, the nurse needs to plan care according to the individual's needs. This can be illustrated using the simple example of dietary needs: a small amount of food, pleasantly presented, may be vital to encourage eating in the elderly patient who has a depressed appetite after surgery. On the other hand, an energetic, young, post-operative patient may require a bulkier dietary intake, while a patient with a learning disability may need reminding of what and when to eat following surgery.

3 *implementation.* In the nursing process, implementation refers to putting into action the interventions planned in the previous stage. From a homeostatic perspective this is analogous to the activation of effector organs to produce an appropriate response.

4 *evaluation.* The effectiveness of perioperative care is assessed in this stage, just as feedback processes provide a means of evaluating a psycho-physiological response. For example, has the injection begun to prevent the patient's pain?

5 *reassessment.* This stage is essential since revised care plans may be considered. This stage emphasizes the cyclical nature of the nursing process. The dynamism of this process is also observed in homeostatic mechanisms described in this book; parameters constantly fluctuate within their normal ranges and such changes perioperatively must, therefore, be constantly reassessed.

(a)

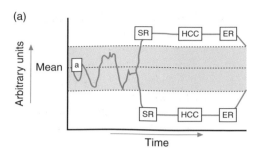

a – Homeostatic dynamism reflecting individual variability,

SR – Receptors detect deviations from the homeostatic range,

HCC – Homeostatic control centres analyse the deviation and its magnitude of change,

ER – Effectors correct the imbalance

(b)

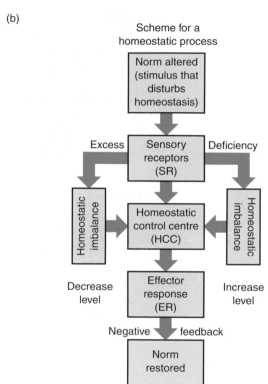

Figure 1.9 **Homeostasis. Control, perioperative intervention illness and nursing process**
(a) and (b): General scheme demonstrating the role of receptors, homeostatic control centres and effectors via negative feedback in a control process. Homeostatic control components.
(See text, pp. 19–22, for details.)

(c)

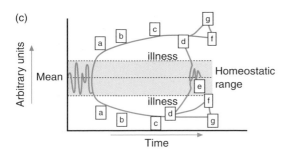

a failure of short-term homeostatic control mechanisms

b failure of intermediate-term homeostatic control mechanisms

c failure of long-term homeostatic control mechanisms

d successful perioperative intervention to re-establish patient homeostasis. For example, surgery to remove diseased tissue or caesarean section. In both cases the homeostatic control centres are unable to respond to correct the homeostatic imbalance and without surgical intervention death would probably occur

e patient's homeostatic status restored

f partially successful perioperative intervention improves quality of life without re-establishing homeostasis

g death – an inability to survive the homeostatic imbalance. For example, the demands of anaesthesia and surgery can cause a failure of the body systems and the perioperative team are no longer able to maintain the homeostatic controls

(d)

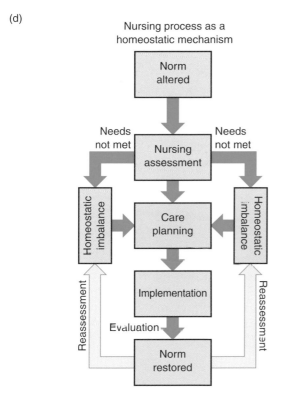

Figure 1.9 Continued
(c): Perioperative interventions following homeostatic control system failure
(d): The nursing process as a homeostatic mechanism (see text pp. 22–3 for details)

Q. Describe the function of the components of homeostatic control when there is a deviation in a parameter being monitored

Q. What do you understand by the statement that perioperative practitioners are external agents of homeostatic control?

EXERCISE

Reflect on your understanding of how lung and kidney function may be affected in a patient who has experienced a myocardial infarction.

Summary

- Humans are biological beings. The biological construction (anatomy and physiology) of the individual provides the basis for identifying how interactions with the external environment influence the psycho-physiological health of the individual.
- The maintenance of bodily functions regulate appropriate cellular activities, which are determined by enzymes, the products of gene expression.
- The composition of the intracellular environment will influence the efficiency with which cells operate, which is why optimal regulation is vital.
- The concept of homeostasis helps to explain the importance to health of maintaining an optimal environment within which cells must function. 'Optimal' does not necessarily equate with constancy. It also relates to the control of change observed during daily activities of living, times of stress, illness and during the perioperative period and the developmental phases of the lifespan.
- Homeostatic control relies mainly upon negative feedback mechanisms that act to reverse changes and regulate parameters close to the optimal value.
- Prevention of parameter variation can be detrimental under some circumstances. The promotion of change via positive feedback mechanisms or through a resetting of homeostatic set-points is then of benefit.
- Ill-health may require surgical intervention when there is a failure to maintain homeostatic functions, either at tissue or organ levels of organization. The interdependency of tissue functions means that those homeostatic disturbances and associated signs and symptoms might also arise secondarily to the primary disorder.
- Perioperative interventions are largely concerned with supplementing normal anatomical, biochemical and hence physiological processes in order to re-establish the homeostatic status of the individual. Therefore, homeostasis provides a working framework for health, and a framework upon which perioperative care should be based.

Bibliography

Campbell, C. and Taylor, M. (1999) Back to basics: the multi-disciplinary team in the operating department. *British Journal of Perioperative Nursing* 9(4): 178–184.

Campbell, C. and Taylor, M. (1999) Back to basics: patient care in the operating department. *British Journal of Perioperative Nursing* 9(6): 272–275.

Cannon, W. (1932) *The Wisdom of the Body*. New York: Norton.

Clancy, J. and McVicar, A.J. (2002) *Physiology and Anatomy. A Homeostatic Approach, Second Edition*. London: Arnold.

This text will expand on many of the physiological principles discussed in this book.

Clancy, J. and McVicar, A.J. (eds). (1998) *Nursing Care. A Homeostatic Casebook*. London: Arnold.

This casebook explores many conditions that require surgical intervention.

Darovic, G.O. (1999) Critical care. Shades of grey: understanding chest x-rays. *Nursing* 28(7): 32.

This article looks at what to look for in x-rays and how to interpret what you see.

Henderson, V. (1996) *The Nature of Nursing*. London: Collier Macmillan.

Kenneth, N., Anderson, K.N. and Anderson, L. (1998) *Mosby's Pocket Dictionary of Medicine, Nursing and Allied Health, Third Edition*. London: Mosby.

This pocket dictionary of medicine, nursing and allied health is an excellent pocket-sized dictionary with strong emphasis on nursing and allied health terminology.

Laudicina, P.F. (2000) Head trauma. *Seminars in Radiologic Technology* 8(1): 7–11, 24–9.

This article discusses the advantages and disadvantages of plain film versus computer-ized tomographic (CT) imaging.

National Association of Theatre Nurses (2000) *Back to Basics*. Harrogate: NATN.

This book covers the core issues that affect every perioperative practitioner on a daily basis. With topics such as anaesthetic care, hand washing, diathermy and recover-ing patients, this book really covers more that just the basics.

National Association of Theatre Nurses (1997) *Perioperative Video and Teaching Pack*. Harrogate: NATN.

This comprehensive video and teaching pack gives a fly-on-the-wall view of the varied activities of a nurse working in the perioperative department.

Pudner, R. (2000) *Nursing the Surgical Patient*. London: Ballière Tindall.

This book takes a comprehensive, patient-centred approach to the nursing care of patients requiring a wide variety of surgical procedure. The book offers readers cases studies and care plans from which to build their knowledge on surgical care.

Roper, N., Logan, W.W. and Tierney, A. (1990) *The Elements of Nursing, Third Edition*. Edinburgh: Churchill Livingstone.

Answers to multiple choice questions

Q. 2, p. 3

The supine position is associated with the pressure areas identified in List C.

The lateral position is associated with the pressure areas identified in List A.

The prone position is associated with the pressure areas identified in List B.

Q. 3, p. 10

A	B	C	D
3	4	2	1

Q. 6, p. 10

A	B	C	D
3	4	2	1

Chapter 2

The surgical approach and endoscopic procedures

Introduction

A surgical approach is utilized to gain access to the internal tissues and organs. The incision site and size is dictated by the nature of the surgery and the preference of the surgeon. It will vary greatly, but the basics will generally be similar since surgical approaches usually have to first cross through the outer structures of the body. The trauma produced by such 'open' access surgery may be substantive, and this contributes to the stress of surgery. In recent years there has been the development of alternative techniques that entail the use of 'minimal access surgery' for examination and even surgical removal of tissue or repair. Such methods appear to be less traumatic than 'open' approaches and, in view of the negative effects of surgical stress (Chapter 7), are becoming increasingly popular.

Accordingly, this chapter explores the surgical approach from these two perspectives, first by considering issues related to gaining access to tissues and organs in 'open' surgery, and second by considering the uses of endoscopes in 'minimal access surgery'.

'Open' surgery: gaining access

For most specialities, gaining access to deep tissues entails crossing through (1) skin, (2) skeletal muscle, and associated (3) blood vessels and (4) nerves. The process will involve cutting, but will also include the teasing apart of tissue in order to reduce the trauma to the site.

The skin

Anatomy of the skin

The skin consists of two principal parts (Figure 2.1): the inner dermis (derm- = layer) and the outer epidermis (epi- = upon). Below the dermis lies a subcutaneous layer (sub- = below, cutaneous = of the skin), sometimes called the 'superficial fascia' since it also includes part of the connective tissue that covers muscles.

Epidermis

The epidermis is a 'stratified squamous epithelium'. This means that it has a number of layers of simple, flattened (i.e. squamous) cells that sit, ultimately, upon a basement membrane of protein:

- a basal layer (= *stratum basale*) that actually sits on the basement membrane. Other cells within the epidermis are generated from the basal layer, and so this is often referred to as the 'germinal' layer of the skin. Whilst some of the new cells produced by cell division maintain this layer, others ascend toward the surface of the skin and form the following layers.
- a layer of 'prickly'-looking cells (= *stratum spinosum*), lying above the basal layer. The cells here have developed protruberances that interlock with those of neighbouring cells, and this is the start of the formation of a structure that will be tough and durable. Tactile nerve endings, called Merkel's discs, may also be present in this layer.
- a layer of cells that contain granules (= *stratum granulosum*), lying above the stratum spinosum. These cells have begun to flatten and to produce keratohyalin, a substance that will eventually be converted into the tough, waterproofing protein keratin. The compound is stored in the cells and so this layer may be referred to as the 'granular' layer. The nuclei of the cells within the layer begin to degenerate and consequently the cells begin to die.
- a layer of tough, hardened (i.e. cornified; = *stratum corneum*) cells, lying above the granular layer, and at the skin surface. By this time the cells are dead. This layer gives the epidermis the toughness needed to provide a barrier against external physical stresses, and environmental agents such as bacteria and chemicals. The latter include water as the epidermis is now impervious. In adults the epidermis is from 0.5–3 mm thick, depending upon site. This especially relates to the thickness of the cornified layer, and hence to the physical stresses placed on that area of skin, though it generally becomes thinner in elderly people since cell division declines with the ageing process.

There are no blood vessels within the epidermis itself: the outer layers are of dead or dying cells, whereas the demands of the inner layer cells are met by blood vessels within the dermis that extend into the vicinity of the basal layer.

EXERCISE

Which of the following is not a layer of cells within the epidermis?

a The 'prickly' layer.
b The granular layer.
c The dermal layer.
d Stratum corneum.

Box 2.1   Application: epidermal wound healing and skin grafting

The germinal layer of the epidermis undergoes rapid cell division in order to maintain the cornified layer. Being this active means that the epithelium regenerates very quickly if damaged. Wound healing of superficial injury is largely by cell migration from the germinal layer and so there is no need for other cell types to migrate from elsewhere, although lateral migration from adjoining epidermal layers may occur. Superficial wounds to the epidermis therefore heal very quickly, without scarring, and tissue structure is soon reorganized.

Wound healing is considered in detail in Chapter 4.

Split-skin grafting

This entails removal of a section of skin and its transferral to another site (Francis 1998; Donato et al. 2000). It is used when there are areas of denuded skin (e.g. burns), where skin is inadequate to close a wound, or if skin has been removed (e.g. in excision of a tumour).

The graft is obtained from a suitable site using a skin graft knife to remove a very thin strip of skin. The section of skin removed is predominantly epidermis. Remnant germinal cells will re-epithelialize the donor site, although great care must be taken to ensure that the raw, exposed dermis is maintained. The graft is transferred to the graft site, which must have an adequate blood supply to support the transplanted tissue.

Dermis

The dermis is largely composed of connective tissue, including fibres of the proteins collagen and elastin. The collagen fibres provide the skin with durability and elastin gives it elasticity. The orientations of these fibres provide surgical 'guides', but they are not actually visible. They are referred to as 'Langer lines' and surgeons will often make an incision in the axis of the fibres, rather then across them. An initial incision may therefore be stretched to reduce the need to cut further. In this way scarring is reduced, and the dermis is more likely to regain its structure afterwards.

The spaces between the fibres contain many of the structures associated with the skin (Figure 2.1), including blood vessels. In the absence of large amounts of the skin pigment melanin it is the visualization of blood within these vessels that mainly determines the colouration of skin. The following list is an aid to patient assessment.

- The drainage of blood away from the skin in shock causes it to take on a greyish colouration.
- Cyanosis, observed when blood is deoxygenated, can also be observed through skin.

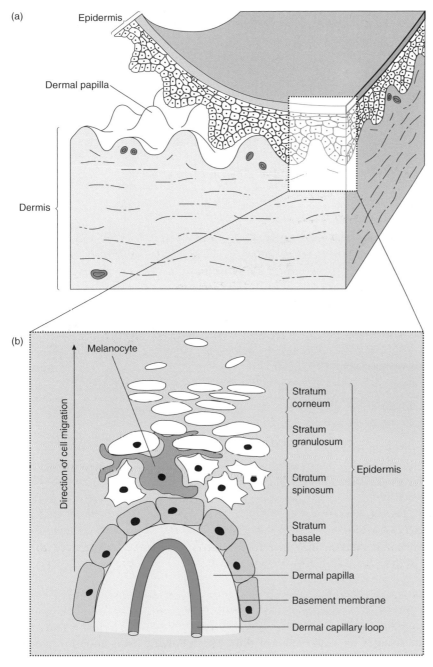

Figure 2.1a **Structure of the skin: the epidermis**
a   General plan and relation to the dermis,
b   Cell layers.

Q. What type of epithelium is the epidermis?

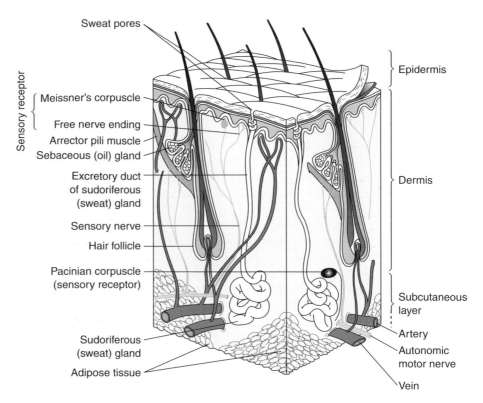

Figure 2.1b **Structures of the dermis and subcutaneous layer**
Note that hairs are epidermally derived and that sweat glands are actually present in the subcutaneous layer. Not shown are the collagen/elastin fibres which form the matrix of the dermis

- The skin will look flushed if the patient is hot as blood flow to the skin is increased.
- The skin circulation is regulated by the sympathetic nervous system, which acts to constrict cutaneous blood vessels, and when this control is inhibited by emotional responses it may even cause 'blushing' as vessels dilate in localized areas.

The dermis also contains many types of sensory nerves and receptors. In fact, the skin is usually viewed as being the largest sensory organ of the body. Senses detected include touch, pressure, temperature ('hot' and 'cold') and pain, and provide information as to what is happening at this interface between the body and external environment.

EXERCISE

Why are the nail beds a good place to observe for cyanosis?

Box 2.2   Application: pressure sores (decubitus ulcers)

A pressure sore is an ulceration of the skin that occurs when there is cell death (necrosis) and tissue atrophy as a consequence of prolonged ischaemia. Pressure sores are commonly observed in people who are immobilized, for example those people perhaps sitting for lengthy spells or confined to bed-rest. Under such circumstances the body weight acts on a point of skin, frequently the buttocks, sacrum or heels, and it is the compression of the skin that induces the ischaemia. The problem is exacerbated if cutaneous circulation is already poor, as in older people or people with diabetes mellitus. In such cases the circulation may be so poor that the skin may even ulcerate without the additional effect of weight.

Preventing the occurrence of ischaemia is an important part of nursing care (Starritt and Ewing 1999). One means of prevention is to reduce the pressure at the interface of the skin and supporting surface. Pressure is minimized by the use of specialized mattresses that incorporate a means of retaining air, or even circulating air, that acts as a cushion for the skin at the point of contact. Other devices may help to regularly move the positioning of the patient and so help to prevent any ischaemia being prolonged. Nurses also have a responsibility to ensure that positioning (either in bed or sitting) does not cause excessive ischaemia.

If ischaemia does occur, and a pressure sore develops, intervention is aimed at maintaining the comfort of the patient (note that the skin is richly endowed with pain receptors), and at promoting wound healing. This latter process can be very slow, however, since granulation of repair tissue is itself dependent upon a reasonable blood supply to the area. The management of such wounds continues to provoke debate, especially in relation to the need to maintain hydration, nutrition and oxygenation of the wound, and of the appropriate dressing type. Interested readers are referred to Harding *et al.* (2000) and Patten (2000).

Subcutaneous layer

This layer attaches the dermis to the underlying tissues (Figure 2.1) and consists of a loose connective tissue, which has relatively few collagen fibres, and of adipose tissue. Loose connective tissue allows laxity of movement of skin across the underlying tissue and this is an aid to the surgeon in exposing the deeper tissues. Also, the presence of loose connective tissue makes this layer an ideal site for injections, since the volume of injectate is more easily accommodated and therefore less painful.

The subcutaneous layer contains two types of gland: the sweat (or sudoriferous) glands and the wax (or ceruminous) glands in the external ear. The ducts of these glands pass to the skin surface via the dermis and epidermis. Sweat, or perspiration, is a mixture of water, salts and products of metabolism (e.g. urea, uric acid, amino acids, ammonia, lactic acid).

■ *Apocrine* sweat glands are found in the skin of the armpits (axillae), pubic areas, and the areolar areas of the breast. Their secretion is viscous because it contains metabolic substances such as fatty acids. These are also useful metabolic substrates for naturally-occurring microbes that reside on the surface of the skin. Replication of such organisms, and the release of microbial secretions, produce 'body odour'.

■ *Eccrine* sweat glands are more widely distributed, though they are absent from lip margins, penis, labia minora and outer ear. They produce a thin, watery secretion, the main role of which is temperature regulation, since the evaporation of eccrine sweat from the body surface has cooling properties.

Box 2.3   Application: paradoxical secretion of sweat in shock

In circulatory shock, sympathetic activity is stimulated by the need to maintain arterial blood pressure whilst cardiovascular functioning is failing (Chapter 5). The symptoms of shock include a cool, pale skin as a consequence of decreased blood supply but the individual will sweat. This is because the sympathetic activity to the skin from the brain that is responsible for the reduction in blood supply simultaneously stimulates the sweat glands. Ordinarily, such outflow would be observed in exercise when losing heat by sweating would be entirely appropriate. In shock, the occurrence of sweating when the skin is cool seems paradoxical and should be recognized as a consequence of impending circulatory failure rather than any need to regulate body temperature.

Perioperative influences on the function of skin

The skin has a number of roles that are compromised by surgery.

Protection

Being in contact with the external environment, the skin is obviously the first line of defence against potential pathogenic organisms. The structure of the skin provides a physical barrier, and the bactericidal constituents of skin secretions also provide a degree of chemical protection against microbes. The impervious nature of skin and its role as a physical barrier also protects the body from chemical agents.

This barrier is breached by surgical procedures, potentially allowing access to underlying tissues for bacteria and other agents. The surgical team reduces the potential for wound infection by (see also Box 4.1):

■ paying attention to the sterility of the theatre environment and implements used.

- wearing sterile overclothes, caps, masks, gloves and theatre shoe's. The hands and arms are thoroughly cleaned pre-operatively using antiseptic skin preparation solutions, such as Betadine™ or Chlorhexadine™.
- by ensuring that the patient has a bath or shower pre-operatively, wears a clean surgical gown, and has clean bed linen.
- by the use of sterile surgical drapes to further protect the patient from infection due to environment contamination.
- by the use of sterile incision drapes to help reduce the risk of wound infection. These drapes stick to the epidermis and reduce the spread of the skin's natural bacteria into the wound. Some surgeons also use incision drapes that are impregnated with iodine solution to help reduce the risk of wound infection.
- reducing the duration of the procedure; the quicker the surgeon, the less time for potential contamination.

Prevention of tissue dehydration

The structure of the intact epidermis makes the skin almost impervious to water. This property of the skin is essential for our existence because it prevents uncontrolled evaporative water loss to the atmosphere. In contrast, surgical procedures, or extensive burns, breach the skin and expose underlying 'wet' tissues to the environment. This could produce extensive loss of water by evaporation, and is a concern for care. Smaller wounds reduce the potential for tissue dehydration, hence the wound should not be extended unnecessarily. Throughout the surgical procedure the use of sterile 'normal' (or isotonic; iso- = equal, tonic- = strength) saline solution to dampen the exposed tissues will also promote the maintenance of tissue hydration.

EXERCISE

How much water is normally lost from the body in twenty-four hours? You might refer to Table 3.2 in considering this.

Regulation of body temperature (thermoregulation)

The surface area of skin in the adult is approximately $1.8\,m^2$ and so provides a major site of heat transfer between the body and external environment. Maintaining an optimal temperature of the essential organs of the body (in this context, the body 'core') is an important aspect of homeostasis, and controlling heat transfer across the skin is part of that regulatory process. Surgery has a number of implications for temperature regulation but first it is important to consider the means by which heat is transferred.

Heat can be transferred to (or in very hot weather from) the environment by three main processes:

1   Radiation. Any physical body at a temperature above absolute zero (0 degrees Kelvin, or –273 °C) will radiate energy. Radiated heat is normally the main way by which heat is lost or gained by the body.
2   Conduction. Conduction is the direct transfer of energy between chemical molecules that have made physical contact with each other. This will include contact between chemicals within the skin and those of air, or of objects in contact with the skin.
3   Evaporation. Converting water into vapour requires energy and so the evaporation of water from the body surface is an effective means of removing heat from the body.

Two fundamental principles operate here:

■   all three routes are unavoidable for the human body,
■   the rate at which heat is transferred by radiation and conduction is determined by the temperature gradient that exists between the skin and external environment.

In order to control the temperature of the body core, therefore, the temperature gradient between the skin surface and environment must be manipulated according to need, and heat loss through evaporation must be regulated (Clancy and McVicar 2002, Chapter 16). Both strategies are employed in health but they are also affected by surgery, and the risk of excessive heat loss is a major concern.

■   *Temperature of the skin.* Physiologically reducing the rate of blood flow to the skin is the main means of reducing the surface temperature, and hence of decreasing heat loss to the environment. Conversely, increasing blood flow to the skin will raise skin temperature and this is a strategy used by the body to promote heat loss in a warm environment. Surgery is unlikely to directly affect these processes but the blood vessels are controlled by sympathetic nerve activity from the brain stem; this is affected by general anaesthetic agents and by responses to trauma, and so the control is unlikely to be as efficient as usual.
■   *Temperature of the environment.* To be precise, it is the temperature of the air or material close to the skin surface that is important here. The presence of insulation material, or the physiological stimulation of piloerection, may trap an unstirred layer of air against the skin; this will form a new immediate environment and will rapidly warm up and so reduce the skin–air temperature gradient. The effect is reduced if convection movements of air around the skin dislodge the unstirred layer, or if the insulation is removed (e.g. changing from everyday clothing to don a theatre gown). Anaesthesia also inhibits the neural pathways that promote piloerection. A better means of producing an appropriate environmental temperature is, of course, to

maintain a suitable ambient temperature. Typically, the operating theatre temperature is maintained at 20–25 °C. This is normally sufficient to promote temperature homeostasis with little need to stimulate physiological mechanisms either to conserve heat or promote its loss. The ambient temperature will be altered as required for the needs of the patient and for the working environment for the surgical team.

■ *Evaporation.* Controlling heat loss through the evaporation of sweat from the skin surface is a vital process for thermoregulation in a warm environment. This effect of evaporation to remove heat from the body is of particular note during surgery because incision of the skin exposes moist tissues and so counters the normal impermeability of skin to water. Water will quickly evaporate from the exposed moist tissues causing cooling (and dehydration).

On balance it is likely that a surgical patient is at risk of losing heat, thus compromising thermoregulation. This potential for excessive heat loss during surgery means that body temperature must be closely monitored during lengthy operative procedures (see Box 2.4).

EXERCISE

Why isn't convection considered to be one of the *primary* routes for heat loss from the body?

Box 2.4   Application: measuring body (core) temperature

The tissues of the body 'core' are accessible by thermometer via the orifices of the body, namely the mouth or nose, external ear (i.e. from close to the ear drum or tympanum, that is, in the vicinity of the brain) and the anus (i.e. from the rectum). When a surgical procedure is expected to take more than 3–4 hours, the patient's body temperature may be monitored using an oesophageal probe; tympanic or (if necessary) rectal probes may be used during the post-operative period. The probes are electrical thermometers: they have a thermistor incorporated into the tip, the electrical resistance of which changes with its temperature (O'Toole 1997). Such thermometers are safer than traditional mercury thermometers since mercury is a toxic metal, and they also produce rapid readings and have good reproducibility (Braun *et al.* 1998).

Note:
■ ear temperatures should be very similar to oral values (a homeostatic range of 36.9–37.1 °C) but values fall sharply and are erroneous if the thermistor is not close enough to the tympanum.
■ rectal temperature is usually slightly higher than the oral value, about 37.5 °C.

Box 2.5   Application: hypothermia in surgery

'Hypothermia' is a core temperature that is below normal homeostatic limits. Neurological and cardiac functions decline with progressive hypothermia, eventually leading to death if the hypothermia is severe. Cold anaesthetic gases, large open body cavities, exposure of body surfaces and the length of the procedure can lower the body temperature, hence control of the patient's body temperature during the perioperative phase is extremely important (McNeil 1998). Patients most at risk are new-born infants, babies and the elderly. Infants and babies have a higher surface area/volume ratio than adults and this facilitates heat loss (since heat loss across the skin relates to surface area, whilst heat generation by metabolism relates to tissue and hence body volume). All three groups have inefficient temperature regulatory mechanisms; in infants and babies the mechanisms are immature (for example, new-born infants cannot shiver) and in older people the efficiency is affected by age-related changes to the capacity for homeostatic control.

Hypothermia can be prevented in a number of ways. An ambient temperature of about 22 °C and a humidity of 55–60 per cent (which reduces rates of evaporation) are recommended in most cases. Cold, dry anaesthetic gases can be supplied through circle systems that absorb carbon dioxide and conserve heat and humidity; heat and moisture exchangers within the breathing circuit can also be used. Conserving heat within body cavities can be achieved by using warm moist gauze packs and warm irrigating fluids. Under-patient heating mattresses, over-blankets that blow warm air over the body surface, and gamgee wrapped around the head and body, all reduce body surface heat loss. Warming devices ensure that all fluids administered intravenously are warm before entering the body. Pre-operatively the patient should be kept warm, and during the post-operative period a warming over-blanket may be necessary.

Beneficial effect of cooling

Sometimes, hypothermia produces such a profound decrease in metabolism that survival may actually be enhanced (being metabolically inactive means that cold tissues become hypoxic much more slowly), and there are numerous instances of apparently 'miraculous' recoveries in people suffering prolonged cold exposure. The principle may be used during surgery. For example, cooling of the heart may be used during coronary bypass surgery, and cooling is used to preserve tissues used for transplantation, since cooling reduces the oxygen demands of tissues and so reduces the risk of damage arising as a consequence of hypoxia caused by disrupted blood supply.

EXERCISE

If body (core) temperature is 37 °C, then why isn't the air temperature of an operating theatre maintained at 30 °C or more in order to prevent the patient becoming hypothermic?

Skeletal muscle

Most skeletal muscles support the skeleton and provide the capacity to move joints, although some are also an integral part of the body wall of the thorax, abdomen and pelvic regions. The extensive distribution of skeletal muscle in the body means surgical procedures are likely to have to cross through muscle at some point.

Skeletal muscle is comprised of muscle fibres; these are functional units of cells that became fused together into a fibre-like arrangement during the differentiation of body tissues (see Clancy and McVicar 2002, Chapter 17). A single muscle fibre may extend along the whole length of a muscle. The advantage of such a structure is that stimulation by associated nerve cells causes entire fibres to contract as if they were each comprised of just one cell, and this makes the contraction of the whole muscle smoother and more rapid than would otherwise be the case. The muscle fibres are found in bunches within the muscle, called fascicles, and are separated from their neighbours by a connective tissue membrane (Figure 2.2). Each fascicle also has an extensive blood supply. The orientation of the fascicles (i.e. of the fibres) determines the direction that a muscle contraction will follow. For example, in the biceps muscle of the upper arm the fascicles are aligned with the longitudinal axis of the muscle, and so when the muscle contracts the forearm is raised towards the shoulder.

Muscles vary considerably in size, depending upon how many fascicles are present, the diameter of individual fibres within the fascicles and the length of the main body of the muscle, called its 'belly'. Muscle strength especially relates to the cross-sectional area of the muscle. Thus, the wide belly of spindle-shaped (or fusiform) muscles such as the biceps are generally able to generate a greater force of contraction than strap types of muscle, such as the rectus abdominis muscle of the anterior abdomen wall. The ends of a muscle usually insert into a skeletal structure via tendons made of dense connective tissue that are continuous with the periosteum, a dense connective tissue that covers the surface of bone.

This complexity of muscle architecture is necessary for their role in providing support for the body and for movement. The tissue is poor at reorganizing itself after injury and so regaining its normal structure (and hence full function) may not be possible. The infiltration of scar tissue into the muscle during wound healing also causes muscle tissue to lose some of its elasticity and contractility. A surgeon therefore will minimize the injury to skeletal muscle during surgery by prising the tissue apart, rather than cutting it (see Box 2.6). The loose connective tissue that forms the fascia over the muscle and around the muscle fascicles will unavoidably be damaged but this usually heals well.

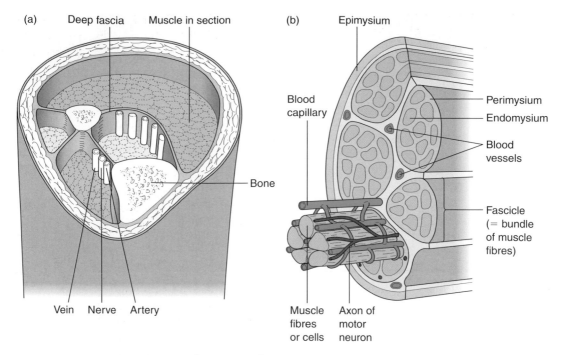

Figure 2.2 **General anatomy of skeletal muscle**
a Whole view in section,
b Detail.

Q. What is the difference between a muscle fibre and a muscle fascicle?

Q. Why does a surgeon prise apart muscles rather than cutting them during the surgical approach?

EXERCISE

Use a suitable anatomy textbook to identify and compare the structure of skeletal muscle and smooth muscle. The latter is found in blood vessels and major organs such as the stomach or colon. As we have noted, surgeons deliberately tease apart skeletal muscle in order to promote a return to function after healing. In contrast, organs such as the colon may be sectioned: how does the structure of smooth muscle facilitate a return to normal functioning of the colon?

Box 2.6   Application: gaining access through muscle

When muscles contract they produce movement along the line of orientation of the muscle fascicles. Surgeons therefore rarely cut laterally through a muscle as this severs the muscle fascicles, though there are exceptions; for example, transverse abdominal incision may be used for emergency access, such as in the repair of aortic aneurysm. Instead they divide the fibres along their length to ensure minimal damage. Where possible, muscle will be left attached to bone but, if it has to be lifted off the bone, enough of the attaching tendon is left to ensure that a suture repair is possible.

A number of muscles arranged in different planes will be involved where multiple ranges of movement are required. For example, the bending, twisting and side-to-side movements produced by the muscles of the abdomen will entail a number of muscles of the abdominal wall.

- *Rectus abdominis*: a pair of long muscles lying medially in the abdomen and extending from the pubic crest of the pelvis up to the rib cage. Contraction of these muscles flexes the vertebral column when we bend over, or may be used to exaggerate movements of the rib cage during forced breathing. The pair of muscles is held together by the fusion of the connective tissue fascia that covers them, which forms a vertical line between the two muscles of toughened tissue called the 'linea alba' (= 'white line').
- *External oblique muscles*: these muscles lie on each side of the rectus abdominis. When one of the muscles contracts it rotates the trunk in one direction; the other muscle produces movement in the opposite direction. The pair contract together to support the rectus abdominis in flexing the vertebral column (and may be used to raise intra-abdominal pressure to aid defecation).
- *Internal oblique muscles*: these muscles lie beneath the external oblique muscles. Their function is similar to those muscles.
- *Transverse abdominis muscles*: these lie beneath the internal oblique muscles. As their name implies, they run more horizontally than do the oblique muscles, and so their contraction causes compression of abdominal organs, for example during defecation.

The surgeon will have to cross through these muscle layers in order to gain access to the abdominal cavity. The rectus abdominis muscles may be separated by an incision made along the linea alba, without incurring blood loss, as the healing qualities of the connective tissue does not impact on the functioning of the muscles themselves. For the other layers of muscle, however, the surgeon will have to work with the various fascicle orientations to prise them apart.

Blood vessels

Blood vessels range from microscopic capillaries to substantial arteries and veins. Blood pressure in the larger arteries is very high (in the aorta it averages 90–95 mmHg), and even within capillaries it is still about 20–30 mmHg, sufficient to cause bleeding if there is trauma. Even in veins, the pressure of a few millimetres of mercury will also cause bleeding if the vessel is punctured. Damage to capillaries and smaller veins, and perhaps to small arteries (called arterioles), is unavoidable during surgery.

Most larger blood vessels share a common basic structure, consisting of three layers or tunicae (= coats). These are described in Chapter 5 but in the context of the surgical approach, the information below should be considered.

- The *tunica interna* consists of a single layer of flattened cells that forms the inner lining of larger vessels. Capillary blood vessels are comprised of this layer only, with little or no elastic fibres, allowing a rapid exchange of water and solutes between the tissue fluid and blood plasma (Chapter 3). This means that there is little elasticity or contractility that might be utilized to stop blood flow from a damaged capillary. However, the vessels are small and are likely to collapse.
- The *tunica media* predominately consists of smooth muscle fibres supported by connective tissue (a layer of collagen and elastin fibres) and is found in arterioles, arteries and veins. This layer therefore has elasticity and contractility. The smooth muscle in the walls of small arteries and arterioles responds to trauma by instantaneously contracting, and this helps to close off the vessel, reduces the blood supply locally, and hence reduces blood loss (Chapter 5).

Nevertheless, seepage of blood is likely to occur. Apart from the problem this introduces of cumulative blood loss over time, the seepage also obscures the surgeon's view. Diathermy (i.e. electrosurgery) may be used to stem the seepage by applying heat that causes blood to clot. Heat may also be used to cauterize the tissue, and so seal the end of small blood vessels (Fullbrook 1998; Wicker 2000). Tying, or ligation, of blood vessels is another method of preventing blood loss.

Large blood vessels normally lie quite deep, though in places such as the wrist they may have to be superficial because of the lack of tissue in these areas. These vessels, when exposed, will normally be left intact during surgery, and only moved aside. If necessary they may be clamped – the muscle and connective tissue in the vessel wall permits them to open up again once clamps are removed.

EXERCISE

A feature of the *tunica interna* is that it is very smooth. What do you think might happen if it was rough, or is roughened by surgical procedures?

Nerves

A nerve is comprised of many nerve cells (or 'neurons') bound together by connective tissue. All neurons contain cell organelles such as a nucleus and mitochondria, but these are largely localized to a 'cell body' and most of what constitutes the neuron is an elongated process (see Clancy and McVicar 2002, Chapter 8). Neurons are classed either as sensory neurons (that convey activity to the spinal cord) or motor neurons (that convey activity away from the spinal cord). The elongated process therefore carries impulses towards the cell body in sensory neurons, since this is located close to the spinal cord, and away from the cell body of motor neurons, since this is located within the spinal cord (Figure 2.3). In sensory neurons the process is referred to as a dendron, and in motor neurons as an axon. These terms are of more interest to students of functional anatomy, and the collective term that is normally applied to the elongated process is 'nerve fibre'. Thus, a nerve is comprised of bundles of nerve fibres, some of which conduct impulses away from the spinal cord, and some of which conduct them to the cord. It is these elongated neuronal cells that are observed albeit microscopically if a nerve is sectioned.

Any loss of neurons will obviously prevent the transmission of neural activity along the usual routes, and so surgeons take care to avoid damage to nerves during the surgical approach.

■   In some cases the nerve will be large enough to be identified and held carefully to one side.

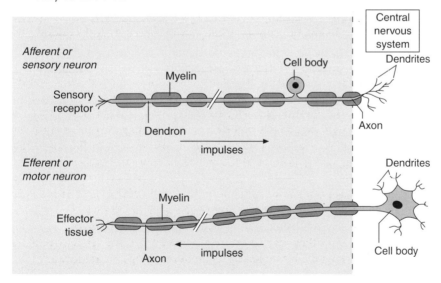

Figure 2.3 **Sensory and motor neurons**

Q. Which part of these cells forms the nerve 'fibre'? What are the dendrites?
Q. What is the role of myelin?

- Similarly, smaller sub-dermal neurons are also avoided if possible, but it is inevitable that some will be damaged. Damaged nerves do have a capacity to repair, utilizing growth factors and chemical attractants to enable the ends of severed fibres to rejoin. Regeneration is very slow, however, and may be incomplete, leaving areas of skin with altered sensory capabilities.
- Damage to receptors and small nerve cells within the skin is minimized by only making a narrow incision in the skin.

Box 2.7   Application: surgery and neural synapses

The text considers trauma to nerve fibres but the operation of nerve terminals may also be influenced by perioperative procedures.

The cell bodies and terminals of nerve cells have extremely fine branching processes. These are essential either because they enable neurons to interact with many other cells in the vicinity, or because the branched endings provide sensory receptors. Where they interact with other cells, actual physical contact between the cells is not usually present, though the 'gap' may only be of the order of 20 nm (20 millionths of a millimetre) wide. The whole structure of the terminal endings and the 'gap' is called a synapse and plays a central role in whether or not nerve impulses are transmitted from one cell to another.

Nerve impulses pass from one cell to another via a process called 'neurotransmission'.

Basically, the nerve impulse stops when it reaches a synapse and has to be regenerated in the succeeding cell(s). This is achieved by the release of a chemical, referred to as a neurotransmitter, that causes a depolarization of the succeeding cell membrane (for a description of depolarization, see Chapter 3). The presence of the synapse is thought to help to prevent onward transmission of any spontaneously generated impulses, since a 'quantum' of activity is required to cause the release of a neurotransmitter in sufficient quantities. The synapse also enables the possibility of opening or closing the route for onward transmission, and so the nerve pathway may be modulated (see the discussion of the 'gate control' mechanism of pain in Chapter 8).

Neurotransmitters

A neurotransmitter will only trigger a nerve or muscle cell if the membrane of that cell has the appropriate receptor sites. This has led to the development of a variety of drugs that can agonize (i.e. activate) or antagonize (i.e. block) the receptors. Each synapse utilizes just one type of neurotransmitter chemical, thus these drugs can be very selective of certain neural pathways. For example, this is the basis for the action of opioid drugs that promote analgesia (Chapter 8) and muscle relaxants that reduce muscle tone and so facilitate the surgical approach (Chapter 7).

EXERCISE

Using an anatomy and physiology text find out why it is essential that a skeletal muscle receives nerve impulses if it is to contract. What is the name of the neurotransmitter that is released at the nerve–muscle synapse?

Minimal access surgery: endoscopy

'Open' surgical procedures may have a major impact on the maintenance of homeostasis, and recovery may take many months. An alternative surgical approach that has a lesser impact on homeostasis is now available for many procedures and is referred to as 'minimal access surgery'. The basic principle here is that access to body cavities is enabled by use of an endoscope (endo- = inside, -scopy = looking) to view internal structures. A light at the tip of the endoscope is used to illuminate the area being investigated and provide a clear view. The image may be transmitted to a TV monitor, or the operator may look directly through the scope.

EXERCISE

In relation to endoscopy, under what circumstances might the following drugs be administered:

a Picolax?
b Midazolam?

The actual equipment used will vary according to the cavity to be examined; the term 'endoscopy' tends to be used in association with the procedure for examining the gastrointestinal tract and specific names are given to other procedures (Table 2.1). This chapter cannot explore all of these types of procedures. Instead it focuses on two in order to illustrate the range of uses of the techniques, and to identify some of the considerations for use. Those discussed are oesophagastroduodenoscopy and laparoscopy.

Table 2.1 Examples of types of endoscopy

Procedure	Organ or tissue visualized
oesophagoscopy	oesophagus
gastroscopy	stomach
duodenoscopy	early duodenum (the first part of the small intestine)
(oesophagastroduodenoscopy)	(a collective term for the above)
colonoscopy	rectum and colon of the large intestine
bronchoscopy	airways: trachea, right and left bronchii
laparoscopy	abdominal cavity
arthroscopy	joint cavity

Q. Through which tissues or structures must an arthroscope be passed?

Oesophogastroduodenoscopy (OGD)

This procedure allows visualization of the oesophagus, stomach and proximal duodenum, the performance of certain surgical procedures and the removal of tissue samples for biopsy. A flexible endoscope (frequently referred to as a 'gastroscope'; gastro- = stomach) is passed via the mouth into the oesophagus, stomach or proximal duodenum. The patient is normally conscious and so patient preparation is extremely important; a full explanation about the procedure should be given as part of the process of obtaining informed consent (British Society for Gastroenterology 1999). The patient must be comfortable during the procedure, and so explanation and reassurance by the perioperative practitioner is vital to keep the patient as relaxed as possible (Panting 1998).

The patient must be starved for a period prior to surgery (see Chapter 3) to facilitate visualization of the stomach and reduce the risk of vomiting during the procedure. To facilitate insertion of the endoscope the patient is placed in the left lateral position, and an intravenous cannula is sited, so that if necessary an intravenous sedative such as Medazolam may be given. A mouth guard is inserted to prevent the patient from biting on the scope, and to protect the teeth. The perioperative practitioner must support the patient's head throughout the procedure as the airway could become compromised. It may also be necessary to use suction to remove excess saliva.

The operator guides the end of a clean endoscope through the mouth, and passes it into the oesophagus as the patient swallows; a local anaesthetic may be applied to the throat to aid tolerance of the endoscope. The passage of the endoscope is monitored. The tip can be bent in several directions, and channels incorporated into the endoscope are used to suction secretions, to flush the tip, and to take samples of tissue for biopsy, as necessary. The endoscope may also be used to dilate constrictions, remove unwanted objects and to arrest bleeding.

Risks associated with OGD

Understandably, OGD risks perforation of the upper gastrointestinal tract and haemorrhage, but the greatest risk to the safety of patients is their reaction to the sedative administered, as this may result in respiratory depression (Cotton and Williams 1996). Resuscitation equipment and antagonist drugs must be readily available. Oxygen therapy may be required if respiratory function is reduced. The patient must be closely observed during the procedure, and vital signs continually recorded to monitor the situation. It is also important to ensure that there is optimal infection control; thorough cleaning and disinfection of the endoscope according to local protocol prior to and after its use is essential.

Recovery of the patient after OGD involves monitoring vital signs, providing advice to the patient, and explaining any side effects of the sedatives used (D'Silva 1998). If a local anaesthetic was applied to the throat then eating and drinking will not be possible until the patient is able to swallow and sensation has returned to the back of the throat.

Examples of applications of OGD

The gastrointestinal tract is essential for ingestion of food (mouth, oesophagus), the digestion or breakdown of complex nutrients (stomach, duodenum, ileum), the absorption of the end products of digestion into the blood (ileum, jejunum) and the elimination of indigestible remains (colon, rectum). Despite having the same basic structure, each part of the tract is specialized for its specific role (Clancy and McVicar 2002; Chapter 10). Accessory organs are also present (for example, the pancreas and liver), which do not come into contact with ingested food, but secrete substances into the tract to aid in digestion and absorption.

EXERCISE

At this point, readers might find it useful to review the structure of the gastrointestinal tract before continuing.

The oesophagus

Examples of disorders of the oesophagus that are diagnosed, and/or treated, using OGD include:

- *oesophageal carcinoma*. A tumour in the oesophagus that is linked with smoking, high alcohol intake and a history of oesophageal trauma or gastro-oesophageal reflux. The majority of tumours appear in the lower two-thirds of the oesophagus.
- *oesophageal varices*. These are often secondary to liver cirrhosis, where weak collateral veins around the oesophagus are distended by the presence of back-pressure from the engorged hepatic portal vein, and can easily rupture. This may lead to large blood loss, and the patient will present with haematemesis or malaena.

The stomach

Common disorders of the stomach that are diagnosed, and/or treated, using OGD include:

- *carcinoma of the stomach*. The majorities of such tumours are located in the pyloric (i.e. lower) region. Patients often present late with anorexia and pain, and generally there is a poor prognosis.
- *gastritis*. This is inflammation of the stomach lining or mucosa, often caused by the ingestion of irritants or some drugs. It has also been linked to chronic alcohol use. It may cause ulceration, and can follow gastric surgery. The patient may present with abdominal pain, vomiting, abdominal distension and anorexia. *Helicobacter pylori* bacteria might be present and can be detected at OGD using a simple test.

■   *ulceration.* The presence in the stomach of strong acid has the potential to erode the mucosal lining. A chronic ulcer may eventually penetrate to the muscular layer of the stomach, where blood vessels may be eroded, causing a significant bleed. Common causes of ulceration are smoking, aspirin or steroid ingestion and stress. Peptic ulcers are also found in the duodenum as a consequence of the acidic chyme that passes into it from the stomach, though usually the duodenum is protected by the neutralizing presence of alkaline digestive juices.

The duodenum

The duodenum is also the location where the bile duct and the pancreatic duct empty into the bowel through the sphincter of Oddi. A form of OGD, referred to as 'endoscopic retrograde cholangiopancreatography' (ERCP), may be used that enables access through this sphincter (see Box 2.8). Common disorders that are diagnosed, and/or treated, using ERCP include:

■   *gallstones.* These can often be undetected, but may cause a partial or complete obstruction of the cystic or common bile duct. Pain, fever and jaundice are common symptoms. The stones normally consist of cholesterol, calcium and bile pigments. Only small stones within the bile duct can be removed using endoscopic methods. Larger stones in the duct or in the gall bladder itself may require abdominal surgery to remove the gall bladder.

■   *pancreatitis.* This is a dangerous inflammatory condition of the pancreas. In severe cases, the digestive enzymes produced by the gland are activated earlier than they should be, within the gland itself, and commence autodigestion leading to oedema, haemorrhage, cell death, disturbances in pH, shock and glucose imbalance. Patients will often present with intense abdominal pain. The most common causes are raised alcohol intake and gallstones that obstruct the common duct.

■   *cancer of the pancreas.* Cancer of the pancreas is usually found in the head region of the organ, close to the duct.

The remainder of the small intestine is comprised of the ileum and jejunum. These sections are too far from the stomach to be accessible by endoscopy, and the highly convoluted nature of the intestine would in any case increase the risk of perforating the bowel wall with the endoscope. New methods are under trial to allow visualization of these segments. At the time of writing a capsule is under test that encloses a miniaturized digital camera, light source and memory chips; this is swallowed by the patient and allowed to progress through the intestine. On recovering the capsule from the colon the images can be downloaded and provide a visual record of the gastrointestinal tract from the mouth to the anus.

The colon itself is accessible using a colonoscope inserted via the anus (see Box 2.9).

Box 2.8   Application: endoscopic retrograde cholangiopancreatography (ERCP)

This procedure employs a side-viewing endoscope so that the sphincter of Oddi, where the common pancreatic/bile duct opens into the duodenum, may be viewed (Bradbury and Bassett 1997; McCormick 1999). ERCP is performed under x-ray, since radio-opaque dye has to be introduced into the duct to locate any blockages. Small stones in the duct can often be removed via this method. A wire is introduced down the endoscope, inserted past the stone, and then a basket or balloon on the end of the wire is opened and the wire withdrawn. This procedure drags the stone out of the duct and into the duodenum, where it can pass through the bowel as normal. If the stone blocks the duct, a sphincterotomy can be performed using the endoscope, where the end of the duct is cut and thus enlarged. Supportive devices called stents may be inserted into either the bile or pancreatic duct to allow free drainage of contents, correcting any narrowing produced by hypertrophy of the duct wall.

In addition to the risks associated with oesophagogastroduodenoscopy (OGD), there is also the potential for ERCP to cause pancreatitis, or infection of the bile duct. However, this procedure can eliminate the need for surgical removal of gallstones by more invasive means using laparotomy (open access to the abdominal cavity) or laparoscopy (endoscopic examination of the abdominal cavity; see text at the bottom of this page).

Box 2.9   Application: colonoscopy

The lower gastrointestinal tract can be examined with a flexible colonoscope through which the whole of the colon can be viewed. Biopsies and the removal of polyps may be carried out using the procedure. The colon must be empty of faeces and bowel preparation may be commenced up to two days in advance, starting with a low residue diet and plenty of water to drink. Picolax may be given the day before to completely clear any faecal residue and an enema may be given on the day of the procedure. For the procedure, the patient is usually placed in the left lateral position and an intravenous cannula sited. Midazolam is commonly used to sedate the patient; opioid pain relief may also be required as air inserted into the colon to aid the view of the colon can cause acute pain and discomfort.

Laparoscopy

Whereas oesophageogastroduodenoscopy, and colonoscopy, utilize an orifice of the body (i.e. the mouth and anus respectively) to access the lumen of the bowel, laparoscopy entails making an access into the abdominal (peritoneal) cavity (Johnson 1999). This technique involves the use of a rigid endoscope (a laparoscope) that is admitted into the peritoneal cavity via a guide inserted into an incision in the abdominal wall. Images transmitted to a TV monitor facilitate the visualization of the peritoneal cavity through the anterior abdominal wall. This procedure is used for both investigative and therapeutic purposes related to the abdominal and pelvic organs (for a history of the development of the procedure, see Spaner and Warnock 1997).

EXERCISE

List the organs of the abdomen that might be accessed by laparoscopy.

The patient is generally placed in a supine position on the operating table, though when pelvic organs are being examined the patient is moved into the Trendlenburg position (see Chapter 1), which causes the abdominal organs to move back under gravity towards the thorax. The entire anterior abdominal wall is prepared from mid-thigh to the nipple line, and also laterally since laparoscopic procedures may occasionally become difficult, necessitating the insertion of additional endoscopic ports away from the original operating site, or conversion to an 'open' procedure (= laparotomy) may become necessary.

The abdominal cavity is initially inflated with gas (producing a 'pneumoperitoneum'; see Box 2.10) to allow the safe introduction of the laparoscope guide, or trocar. The space that is created also improves the visibility of the abdominal contents.

A trocar, covered with a trocar sleeve, is introduced through the abdominal wall into the (inflated) peritoneal cavity. Again the easiest site to insert the trocar is under the sub-umbilical area. The trocar makes a hole in the abdominal wall and the sleeve, referred to as a 'port', remains as a passageway for the laparoscope. The trocar is carefully introduced, generally at a 45° angle facing the pelvic cavity; insufflation may be resumed via the trocar sleeve to maintain abdominal distension. If a blunt port is used for insufflation (see Box 2.10) it is large enough to facilitate the laparoscope and does not need replacing with a larger port. The laparoscope with either a 0° or 30° angle of vision at the tip is introduced into the peritoneal cavity. Additional trocars (for examples see Figure 2.4) may be introduced now under direct vision from the laparoscope so that other instruments can be used to carry out a surgical procedure.

The instruments used are very different from conventional surgical instruments; they are long and slim as they have to pass through ports ranging from just 2 mm to 15 mm in diameter. Instrument length enables the surgeon to reach the abdominal structures, and the instrument is operated from the handle. Any tissue specimens or biopsies can be removed via a port.

Upon completion of the procedure, traces of bleeding are stopped and the laparoscope is withdrawn. The carbon dioxide used to inflate the abdominal cavity is allowed to escape via a port. Any retained gas can cause acute referred pain in the shoulder area, and abdominal discomfort post-operatively.

Once all the trocar sleeves have been removed, the small incisions are closed either by suture or 'steristrips' and dressings. The patient often goes home on the day of surgery or the following day and should return to normal activities within a few days.

Box 2.10   Application: creating a pneumoperitoneum

A pneumoperitoneum is a gas-filled peritoneal cavity that can arise pathologically (Steuer 1998). For laparoscopic investigation the presence of an induced pneumoperitoneum is an advantage because it provides better visualization of the internal organs. This is created by one of two methods.

1 Introducing a (Verres) needle into the peritoneal cavity

The safest access into the intra-abdominal cavity is via the sub-umbilical area because the anterior abdominal wall is thinnest at this level.

The anterior abdominal wall must first be elevated, to distance it from underlying organs, and this is achieved by grabbing the abdominal wall directly under the umbilicus with one hand. A small incision is made and the Verres needle is slowly inserted into the incision, angled toward the pelvis and advanced. If this is done easily and without obstruction, the tip should finish in the proper position. However, the presence of blood or bowel content in the needle means that either a blood vessel or section of bowel has been punctured. Should this occur then it becomes necessary to leave the needle in position and proceed to 'open access' surgery, since to proceed means that there will be a risk of contamination of the peritoneal cavity.

Once in position, the Verres needle is connected to tubing attached to the inflation device, or insufflator. This is switched on and a small amount of carbon dioxide gas admitted into the peritoneal cavity. The entry pressure at this point enables an assessment of resistance to gas flow and is checked immediately while the abdominal wall is still elevated. If it is high then there is probably an obstruction, and so the needle may be manipulated to free the needle tip. The needle might even have to be reintroduced. Once the needle is in a correct position, the intra-abdominal cavity is inflated with about 2–3 litres of CO_2. The gas is introduced until a pre-set desired pressure is reached, when the insufflator automatically modifies the flow to prevent overinflation. The Verres needle is then removed.

2 Applying the 'Hassan' technique

An alternative to the Verre's needle approach, and perhaps a more common approach today, is to use a blunt 10 mm trocar (laparoscope guide) to introduce the gas. An incision is made in the abdominal wall of the sub-umbilical area and the tissue is dissected through the fat, muscle and peritoneal layers. The trocar is then inserted into the peritoneal cavity and sutured into place. CO_2 can then be administered directly into the peritoneal cavity, and the trocar then used to introduce the laparoscope.

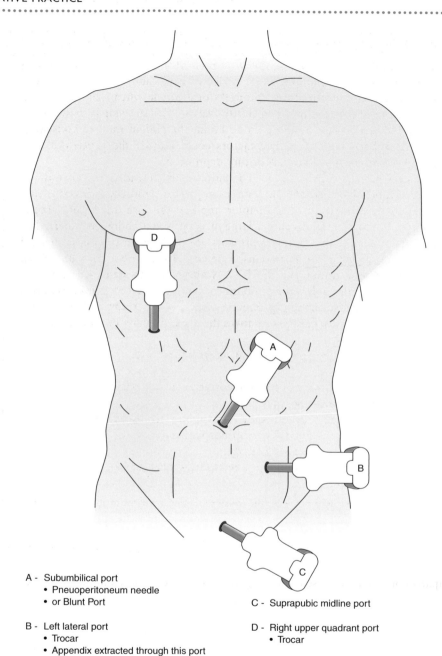

A - Subumbilical port
  • Pneuoperitoneum needle
  • or Blunt Port

B - Left lateral port
  • Trocar
  • Appendix extracted through this port

C - Suprapubic midline port

D - Right upper quadrant port
  • Trocar

Figure 2.4 **Sites for inserting trocars for laparoscopic appendicetomy surgery**

Q. What sort of instruments, other than the laparoscope itself, might be inserted via the trocars?

Box 2.11   Application: advantages and disadvantages of endoscopy

The potential risks of endoscopy have been identified at various points in this chapter. The techniques carry a risk of perforating the tissues, partly because visibility is not always assured (for example when first introducing a verrus needle or trocar), and partly because the surgeon is viewing the tissue indirectly via a monitor. In addition, the patient may be conscious, though sedated, and so patient-factors could impede the procedure. The use of sedation can lead to respiratory depression.

Nevertheless, endoscopy has a number of considerable advantages (Spaner and Warnock 1997). Both examples of endoscopic investigation that are described in this chapter replace the use of 'open access' approaches that entail making a large incision in the abdomen (referred to as 'laparotomy'). Laparotomy represents one of the most traumatic surgical procedures as far as stress responses are concerned (Friedrich *et al.* 1999); it entails major trauma to the body wall simply to gain access to the viscera, and hence substantive wound healing is required. Similarly, open access orthopaedic surgery produces greater tissue trauma than arthroscopy; likewise bronchoscopy removes the need, in many instances, for thoracic surgery.

Important advantages of minimal access surgery are:

- a minimum disruption to the homeostatic controls within the body,
- a reduction in post-operative pain,
- a lower incidence of post-operative respiratory complications,
- a more rapid recovery and shorter hospital stay,
- an earlier return to normal activity,
- less wound complications, e.g. infection and delayed wound healing,
- a better cosmetic effect.

Examples of applications of laparoscopy

Laparoscopy may be used for diagnostic purposes, for example to look for lesions, adhesions or growths that might explain the occurrence of abdominal pain. It may also be used for surgical removal of tissue, or for repair. Tissues removed or treated surgically relate to most of those organs that are accessible within the abdominal cavity. Surgical procedures commonly undertaken by laparoscopy include:

- *cholecystectomy:* removal of the gall bladder, perhaps because of extensive stone formation.
- *urolithectomy:* removal of stones from within the kidney.
- *nephrectomy:* removal of a kidney, perhaps because of the presence of a tumour.

- *hysterectomy*: removal of the uterus, perhaps because of the presence of a carcinoma.
- *oophrectomy*: removal of an ovary, perhaps because of an ovarian cyst or tumour.

EXERCISE

Laparoscopic surgery has a number of advantages (see Box 2.11) but also introduces risks. For example, read the article by Terpestra (1996) on the application of laparoscopy to cholecystectomy.

Summary

- Open access surgery requires the surgical approach to incise or cross through various tissues.
- The protective barrier that is formed by the skin is breached by an incision, with potential risks for infection, dehydration and hypothermia.
- The surgical approach minimizes damage by using the natural elasticity of skin tissue to expand an incision without the need for further cutting.
- Similarly, muscle fibres are usually separated, rather than cut, as this facilitates wound healing without excessive scarring.
- Whenever possible, nerves and large blood vessels are moved to one side. However, damage to small nerves and vessels is unavoidable and steps will be taken to minimize bleeding, using diathermy, sutures or clamps as appropriate. Damaged nerves may regenerate some time after surgery but this may be incomplete.
- 'Minimal access surgery' uses endoscopes to examine internal cavities and tubular structures. The scopes contain a light source and, via fibre optic connections, enable images to be produced on monitors.
- Various procedures are employed depending upon the tissue under examination.
- Oesophagogastroduodenoscopy enables examination of the upper gastrointestinal tract. The method is especially useful for investigative procedures where growths, erosions or blockages are anticipated. The technique allows some operative procedures to be performed that otherwise would have required open access.
- Laparoscopy enables examination and operative procedures of the abdominal cavity. The incisions that are required to insert the laparoscope and supportive instruments are minimal.
- In many instances endoscopy removes the need for open access surgery, and so minimizes the tissue trauma, risk of infection, dehydration and hypothermia. Wound healing is faster, recovery is quicker and cosmetic effects are also more favourable. The advantages are therefore extensive, though the procedures do have risks.

Bibliography

Bradbury, M. and Bassett, C. (1997) Medical investigations: principles and nursing management. *Medical investigations 2: ERCP. British Journal of Nursing* 6(8): 460–1.

Braun, S.K., Preston, P. and Smith, R.N. (1998) Getting a better read on thermometry. *Registered Nurse* 61(3): 57–60.

British Society for Gastroenterology (1999) *Guidelines for Informed Consent for Endoscopic Procedures.* London: British Society for Gastroenterology.

Champion, J. (2000a) Risk assessment: a five step process. *British Journal of Perioperative Nursing* 10(7): 350–3.

Champion, J. (2000b) Laser safety management. *British Journal of Perioperative Nursing* 10(8): 428–32.

Clancy, J. and McVicar, A. (2002) *Physiology and Anatomy: A Homeostatic Approach.* London: Arnold.

Copeland, S. (1998) Arthroscopy and arthroscopic surgery of the shoulder. *British Journal of Perioperative Nursing* 8(3): 5–10.

Cotton, P. and Williams, C. (1996) *Practical Gastrointestinal Endoscopy. Fourth Edition.* Oxford: Blackwell Science.

Dennison, R.D. (1997) Nurse's guide to common postoperative complications. *Nursing* 27(11): 56–9.

Donato, M.C., Novicki, D.C. and Blume, P.A. (2000) Skin grafting: historical and practical approaches. *Clinics in Podiatric Medicine and Surgery* 17(4): 561–98.

D'Silva, J. (1998) Upper gastrointestinal endoscopy: gastroscopy. *Nursing Standard* 12(45): 49–54.

Francis, A. (1998) Nursing management of skin graft sites. *Nursing Standard* 12(33): 41–4.

Friedrich, M., Rixecker, D. and Friedrich, G. (1999) Evaluation of stress-related hormones after surgery. *Clinical & Experimental Obstetrics & Gynecology* 26(2): 71–5.

Fullbrook, S. (1998) A nurse's scope of practice, control and diathermy in the operating department. *British Journal of Perioperative Nursing* 8(1): 39–42.

Harding, K., Cutting, K. and Price, P. (2000) The cost-effectiveness of wound management protocols of care. *British Journal of Nursing* 9(19) Supplement S6–S27.

Johnson, A. (1999) Laparoscopic surgery. *British Journal of Perioperative Nursing* 9(3): 119–24.

Kent, S. (2000) Antiseptic skin preparation revisited. *British Journal of Perioperative Nursing* 10(7): 364–72.

McCormick, M.E. (1999) Endoscopic retrograde cholangiopancreatography. *American Journal of Nursing* 99(2): 24HH–JJ.

McNeil, B. (1998) Addressing the problems of inadvertent hypothermia in surgical patients Part 1: addressing the issues. *British Journal of Perioperative Nursing* 8(4): 8–18.

O'Toole, S. (1997) Alternatives to mercury thermometers. *Professional Nurse* 12(11): 783–6.

Panting, A. (1998) Preparing patients for endoscopy. *Nursing Times* 94(27): 60.

Patten, J. (2000) A case study in evidence-based wound management. *British Journal of Nursing* 9(12) Supplement S38–S49.

Scott, E. (1998) Hospital-acquired pressure sores as an indicator of quality: a research programme centred in the operating theatre. *British Journal of Perioperative Nursing* 8(5): 15–18.

Spaner, S.J. and Warnock, G.L. (1997) A brief history of endoscopy, laparoscopy, and laparoscopic surgery. *Journal of Laparoendoscopic & Advanced Surgical Techniques. Part A.* 7(6): 369–73.

Starritt, T. and Ewing, E. (1999) Implementing good practice in the prevention and management of pressure sores. *British Journal of Perioperative Nursing* 9(2): 60–3.

Steuer, K. (1998) Pneumoperitoneum – physiology and nursing interventions. *AORN Journal* 68(3): 410–26 [erratum *AORN J* (1999) 69(1): 21].

Terpestra, O.T. (1996) Laparoscopic cholecystectomy: the other side of the coin. Choose between a larger scar or a slightly larger risk of bile duct injury. *British Medical Journal* 312(7043): 1375–6.

Waterlow, J. (1996) Operating table: the root of many pressure sores? *British Journal of Theatre Nursing* 6(7): 19–21.

Wicker, P. (2000) Electrosurgery in perioperative practice. *British Journal of Perioperative Nursing* 10(4): 221–6.

Woollons, S. (1996) Temperature measurement devices. *Professional Nurse* 11(8): 542–7.

Chapter 3

Perioperative influences on body fluid homeostasis

Introduction

The adult body contains approximately 40–45 litres of water, equivalent to 60–65 per cent of body weight. This substantial volume provides more than a body 'filler': it supports tissues, enables the circulation of nutrients, and is the medium in which most if not all biochemical reactions take place. Fluid distribution and composition is therefore important and body fluid homeostasis must ensure that this volume and composition is conducive to optimal cell and tissue functions. Surgery has potentially major implications for the maintenance of body fluid homeostasis because of the practice of fasting patients preoperatively, of the surgical procedure itself, the responses to trauma, or the incidence of post-operative complications.

This chapter explains the basic physiology of body fluid maintenance, and explores how surgery influences fluid homeostasis. The rationale for the choice of intravenous fluid for administration is also described. Before proceeding, however, it is worth noting how osmosis operates, since this is the main process that ensures the distribution of water within the body.

Osmosis

Osmosis is defined as the movement of solvent (i.e. water) across a selectively permeable membrane from a solution of low solute concentration to one of a higher concentration. The process is illustrated in Figure 3.1. From this diagram, it can be seen that osmosis is actually a special form of diffusion, because it relates to the movement of solvent molecules themselves rather than molecules of dissolved substances, or solutes.

The direction and rate of movement of water molecules will depend upon the concentration of dissolved solute on each side of a selectively permeable membrane since this determines the relative number of water molecules present per

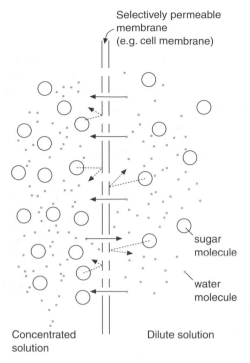

Figure 3.1 **Movement of water molecules by osmosis**

Q. What would happen if the membrane was permeable to the sugar molecules?

unit of volume. For example, a millilitre of a strong sugar solution will contain fewer water molecules than a millilitre of a more dilute sugar solution, as the sugar molecules will occupy more space. If a membrane that is impermeable to the sugar molecules, but is permeable to water molecules, separates the two solutions, then water will pass by osmosis into the strong solution. The strong sugar solution therefore is said to have a greater osmotic 'potential' than the dilute solution.

In a laboratory experiment it might be possible to apply a pressure to the strong solution which will prevent the osmosis from occurring (as pressure will tend to force the water molecules back across the membrane). The degree of pressure that has to be applied will equate with the osmotic potential and so the terms 'osmotic potential' and 'osmotic pressure' are both used in relation to osmosis. In practical terms, osmotic pressure is difficult to measure and the osmotic potential must be assessed by different means. This is done by determination of the effect that the dissolved solutes have to depress the freezing point of the solution. In the example of sugar solutions, the freezing point depression will be greater for a strong solution than it is for a weaker one. The value is converted to an 'osmolality', with the units 'milliosmoles per kg of water' (this approximates to 'milliosmoles per litre' for the range of solute concentrations in body fluids). It is this value that may appear on blood analyses; the solutes dissolved in plasma give it a normal osmolality of about 285 milliosmoles per kg of water.

'Osmotic potential', 'osmotic pressure' and 'osmolality' are all used in the literature to describe the solute concentration of a solution. Whilst this may seem confusing, they are generally interchangeable in this respect. However, the context in which they are used is also important. This is especially appropriate for osmotic pressure where it applies to the exchange of water between blood capillaries and the fluid bathing the tissues since this exchange is determined by the imbalance in pressures across the capillary wall, as is explained later.

EXERCISE

Seawater contains minerals found in body fluids. Why then are we unable to drink it?

Body fluids and their distribution

Water is not evenly distributed throughout the body. Of the 40–45 litres of water present in the adult, approximately 25 litres are found within cells, and so comprise an intracellular fluid compartment (intra- = inside), and the remainder is found outside the cells, and so comprises an extracellular compartment (extra- = outside).

Extracellular fluid compartment

The extracellular fluid compartment is sub-divided into three sub-compartments (Figure 3.2).

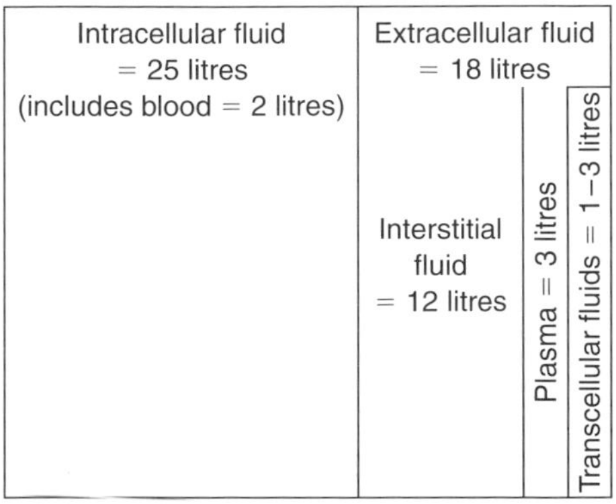

Figure 3.2 Body fluid compartments and their volumes (adult)

Q. Can you provide four examples of a transcellular fluid?

Interstitial, or tissue, fluid

This is the component that bathes most of our cells and has a volume (in adults) of approximately 12 litres.

Blood plasma

This is the fluid component of blood in which blood cells are suspended, and in an adult has a volume of approximately 3 litres. It corresponds to the tissue fluid of blood, but is considered separately. Nevertheless, plasma is in continuity with tissue fluid throughout the body and most of their constituents actually exchange, as identified below.

Transcellular fluids

These are specialized extracellular fluids, such as the cerebrospinal fluid (CSF), gastrointestinal fluid and intraocular fluid, that are not continuous with either blood plasma or tissue fluids. These fluids are secreted by layers of cells that form a barrier between them and other extracellular fluids, although ultimately they must be derived from blood plasma. Collectively they have a volume of approximately 1–3 litres: their total volume varies according to the volume of fluid that is secreted, especially in the bowel. Individually, their volume and composition may be very closely regulated, for example, the volume of CSF hardly varies. This is vital to the functioning of the specific tissue with which they are associated. Disorders of their regulation can have widespread consequences; for example, note the effects of excessive peritoneal fluid (see Box 3.2) and pleural fluid (Chapter 6) but generally these are considered as individual, special cases and so are not discussed further in this chapter.

EXERCISE

Where in the body would you expect to find the following transcellular fluids?

a   cerebrospinal fluid.
b   gastric fluid.
c   synovial fluid.
d   intrauterine fluid.
e   intraocular fluid.

Which is likely to have the largest volume?

Regarding extracellular fluid, the main distinction is between tissue fluid and blood plasma. The distribution of these fluids is determined by the exchange that occurs within the capillary beds of tissues. Pores in the membranes of capillary blood vessels permit the passage of small solutes such as electrolytes and glucose, but protein molecules found in abundance in plasma are too large to cross; thus it is a selectively permeable membrane (see 'Osmosis', above, p. 57). The protein concentration in plasma is considerably higher than it is in tissue fluid, and this differential is sufficient to favour movement of water from the tissue fluid into the plasma. This effect of plasma proteins is referred to as the 'colloid osmotic pressure' (see Box 3.1) but it is counteracted by the hydrostatic pressure within the blood vessels. Although blood pressure within capillaries is much less than it is in arteries (the capillaries are much more delicate), it is sufficient early in the capillary to exceed the colloid osmotic pressure and so water and its solutes (except protein) pass from the plasma into the tissue fluid (Figure 3.3). The loss of fluid from plasma means that the blood pressure falls along the capillary, and a point is reached where it no longer exceeds the colloid osmotic pressure, eventually falling below it whence fluid is drawn back into the capillary from the tissue fluid.

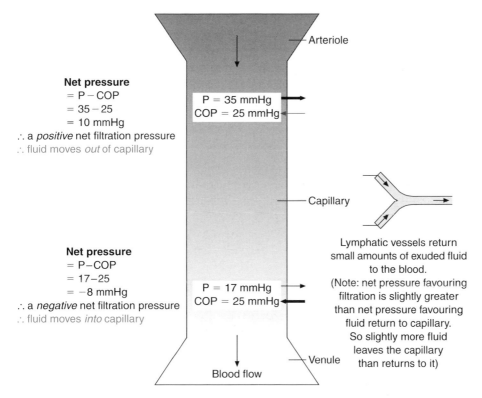

Figure 3.3 **Capillary exchange: forces influencing fluid movement between plasma and tissue fluid**

P = (Blood) pressure within the capillary. This decreases along the capillary as fluid leaks out.

COP = Colloid osmotic pressure due to plasma proteins.

Q. Why does blood pressure within the capillary decrease on passing from the arteriolar to the venous ends?

> ### Box 3.1 Application: colloid osmotic pressure and crystalloid osmotic pressure
>
> Proteins and protein substitutes are large molecules that form a viscous, sticky solution when dissolved in water. They are referred to as 'colloids' since they form this suspension-like solution. In contrast, substances such as glucose and electrolytes are fully soluble in water and are referred to as 'crystalloids' (both glucose and salts form crystals when dried).
>
> Both types of solute will promote osmosis if there is an effective solute gradient. Considering body fluids in general, the osmotic potential is primarily due to the dissolved crystalloids and it is these solutes that together determine the movement of water across cell membranes by osmosis. However, the colloids are extremely important in relation to capillary exchange since these blood vessels are fully permeable to the crystalloid solutes and so it is the colloids (i.e. proteins) in plasma that are most effective at capillary level. Capillary exchange is explained in the text.

The interplay between the capillary blood pressure and osmosis due to plasma proteins ensures that nutrients in plasma are delivered into the vicinity of cells within the tissues, and excess and 'wastes' or secretions from cells are efficiently returned to blood. The forces are closely matched, and so almost the same volume of water is returned to the capillary as was lost from it. Consequently, the volume of blood leaving the capillary to enter the venous system is maintained, and the accumulation of fluid within tissues is prevented. In reality, the forces are not exactly balanced, and a small net loss of water into the tissue fluid does occur. This small excess is returned to the blood via lymphatic drainage from the tissues. This is actually of advantage to the body since lymph passes through lymph nodes before returning to the blood, hence the presence of any infectious agent within the tissues can be intercepted (Chapter 4),

> ### Box 3.2 Application: influence of surgery on the distribution of extracellular fluids
>
> *Oedema*
>
> Reference to Figure 3.3 will aid the interpretation of the following.
> Oedema is an accumulation of tissue fluid and will arise when:
>
> - capillary blood pressure is elevated above normal since this favours the discharge, or exudation, of fluid from plasma. This usually occurs if venous pressure is elevated; the presence of 'resistance' vessels (i.e. arterioles) between arteries and capillaries prevents oedema when arterial blood pressure is increased. The oedema may be localized, for example swollen ankles on a hot day, or generalized, for example in congestive heart failure.

- blood plasma becomes deficient in protein, thus reducing the osmotic pressure of the plasma. This normally arises either because protein synthesis has been reduced (e.g. in liver failure), or because protein has been excreted in the urine (e.g. in glomerulo-nephritis). The oedema is usually generalized.
- lymphatic drainage from tissues is obstructed because the tissue has been compressed or traumatized. This is usually localized to the area affected.
- capillary membranes leak protein into the tissue fluid, resulting in a localized reduction in plasma protein concentration. This is frequently very localized, for example during an inflammatory response to infection.

Oedema may occur during the perioperative period. Localized oedema may arise when interrupted lymphatic drainage occurs when flaps of tissue are turned aside, or because of an inflammatory response to tissue damage. Both may hinder the repair of a wound (Hofman *et al.* 1998). Localized oedema may also arise if there is partial occlusion of wound drainage, leading to accumulation of discharged fluid, or exudate; the risk here is of altered wound healing, or even the development of ulceration in the area. Most serious is the risk of pulmonary oedema as a consequence of an inflammatory response in the alveoli, for example in pneumonia or in acute respiratory failure (see Chapter 6).

'Third space syndrome'

Major surgery may cause a rapid shift in the distribution of extracellular fluid. Thus:

- increased sympathetic nerve activity as a result of stress responses (Chapter 7) or low blood pressure (Chapter 5) may cause the bowel to cease contracting, producing 'paralytic ileus'. A potential problem here is that the bowel will continue to produce its secretions but these will not be passed along the ileum and so will not be reabsorbed.
- peritonitis may lead to an increased permeability of the peritoneum and hence to the rapid accumulation of fluid within the abdominal cavity. This is a form of oedema called ascites.

Under either of these circumstances the loss of fluid from the plasma and tissue fluid might be as much as several litres per day, thus increasing the risk of hypovolaemia and hence hypovolaemic shock. This effect is sometimes referred to as 'third space syndrome' because its occurrence makes it appear that a third major fluid compartment has suddenly become available.

> **EXERCISE**
>
> Why do people's ankles sometimes swell in hot weather?

Intracellular fluid compartment

The intra- and extracellular compartments are separated by the cell membrane, which is mainly comprised of lipid derived from cholesterol. Many substances are found within the body fluids that will dissolve in water but not in lipid. For example, glucose is very soluble in water but it is so poorly soluble in lipid that it cannot simply diffuse into cells. The cell membrane therefore provides a degree of isolation of the two fluid compartments, and therefore facilitates the maintenance of an intracellular fluid that has a different composition to that of the extracellular fluid (Table 3.1). Cells require many substances to cross the cell membrane, for example glucose is required for energy (Chapter 7), and this means that the cell membrane must contain mechanisms to enable this to occur. There are structural proteins within the membrane that provide pores or perhaps carriers for substances, which are under the control of the cell. The extent of this control is such that the pores or carriers are highly selective, providing a means of entrance/exit for just one substance, such as a specific ion (see Box 3.4 for an example). By controlling the 'opening' or 'closing' of the pores, or the presence and/or activity of the carriers, the cell membrane is able to regulate the movement of substances into and out of the cell.

Table 3.1 Composition of intracellular and extracellular fluids

Constituent	Extracellular fluid		Intracellular fluid
	Plasma (mmol/l)	Tissue fluid (mmol/l)	Skeletal muscle cell (mmol/l)
Cations			
Sodium Na$^+$	142	145*	12
Potassium K$^+$	4.3	4.4	150
Calcium Ca^{2+}	1.2**	1.2**	4
Anions			
Chloride Cl$^-$	104	117*	4
Bicarbonate HCO^{3-}	24	27*	12
Phosphate HPO$_4^{2-}$; H$_2$PO$_3$	2	2	40
Proteins	70 g/l	Approx. 0	25 g/l
pH	7.4	7.4	7.0

Note
*Slight differences from plasma arise because plasma proteins are negatively charged and this interferes with ion diffusion.
**Ionized calcium. Approximately the same amount is bound to proteins.

In contrast, water molecules are able to move freely in and out of cells. Therefore they will cross by osmosis if a solute concentration gradient is present. However, this will relate to the *total* concentration of solute inside and outside cells, and the differential composition in Table 3.1 has no consequence. But if the total concentration should change, increased for example because of dehydration of the extracellular fluid, then osmosis will occur. In dehydration, water will move out of the cells until a new equivalence occurs between the intra- and extracellular fluids. Dehydration therefore results in an elevated solute concentration both inside and outside cells, and a reduced volume of both compartments. The reduced volume of intracellular fluid disrupts the appearance of cells; the cells assume a 'crinkled' appearance referred to as 'crenation'. This, coupled with the altered composition of the intracellular fluid, compromises cell functioning. Similarly, overhydration lowers the concentration of solutes in both compartments by promoting osmosis into the cell. In this instance cell volume increases; if the overhydration is very severe then the cells might even burst (a process called '-lysis', e.g. haemolysis is the bursting of red blood cells).

Box 3.3   Application: turgor pressure

Turgor is the hydrostatic pressure that is exerted by intracellular and tissue fluids, and helps to maintain the firmness of the tissue. For example, if we pinch a small area of well-hydrated skin it feels firm and quickly springs back into position. If an individual is very dehydrated then the skin feels less resistant and returns to its original position much more slowly. Loss of turgor is most apparent from areas where the skin is quite thin since there is less connective tissue to support it, for example around the eyes where dehydration produces a 'sunken' appearance. The loss of skin elasticity with age means that turgor is less readily assessed in older people.

Electrolyte composition of intracellular and extracellular fluids

What are electrolytes?

'Electrolyte' is another term for an ion, which is a form of an atom that carries an electrical charge because it has either gained or lost electrons from its atomic structure. Electrons are negatively charged particles and so those atoms that gain one or more electrons become negatively charged, and are referred to as anions, whilst those that lose electrons are positively charged and called cations. A salt consists of a cation and an anion joined together. For example:

$$\begin{array}{ccc} \text{NaCl} & \longrightarrow & \text{Na}^+ \;+\; \text{Cl}^- \\ \text{sodium chloride} & & \text{sodium} + \text{chloride} \\ \text{i.e. salt} & & \text{cation} + \text{anion} \end{array} \qquad (3.1)$$

The presence of an electrical charge means that solutions of ions are able to conduct an electrical current, and this is indicated by the term 'electrolyte'.

EXERCISE

Regarding the number of electrons found in ions, how does a sodium ion differ from:

a a sodium atom?
b a chloride ion?

Hydrogen ions and bases

Hydrogen ions are produced by acids: they are the smallest possible ions and are extremely reactive. In cells they have the potential to disrupt biochemical reactions, primarily because they cause protein structures to alter their shape. This particularly affects those proteins, or enzymes, that are essential because they speed-up chemical reactions in cells (referred to as catalysts).

Hydrogen ions are produced when an acid dissociates in water. For example, hydrochloric acid dissociates into hydrogen and chloride ions:

$$HCl \rightleftharpoons H^+ + Cl^-$$

Hydrochloric acid   Hydrogen ion   Chloride ion   (3.2)

This is analogous to equation 3.1 in that a cation (i.e. hydrogen) and an anion (chloride) is produced. Unlike salts, however, acids are not found in a solid state when they are not dissolved in water (they are usually formed from a reaction between a gas and water). Nevertheless, hydrogen ions are positively charged and so are considered to be cations. The chloride ion is an anion, but in the context of being able to combine with hydrogen ions in this reaction is also referred to as a 'base'. Thus, a base is a chemical that will combine with hydrogen ions to form an undissociated (acid) molecule.

In equation 3.2, the hydrogen and chloride ions will recombine to form hydrochloric acid. This is a 'strong' acid and the acid molecules will immediately dissociate again. As a consequence, at any given moment in time the solution will be comprised almost entirely of hydrogen and chloride ions. In contrast, some acids do not dissociate easily and are 'weak' acids. For example, carbon dioxide combined with water produces carbonic acid:

$$CO_2 + H_2O \rightleftharpoons H_2CO_3 \rightleftharpoons H^+ + HCO_3^-$$ (3.3)

carbon   water   carbonic   hydrogen   bicarbonate
dioxide   acid   ion   ion

Once again the reaction is reversible and so acid will reform. In this instance, the tendency for carbonic acid to dissociate is very weak, and so at any moment in time the reaction favours the formation of acid molecules, thus the concentration of hydrogen ions in the solution will be low, though some will be present.

The amount of hydrogen ions in a solution could be measured directly in terms of the hydrogen ion concentration, but conventionally is measured in pH units:

pH1 $\longleftarrow$ pH7 $\longrightarrow$ pH14

strong   weak   weak   strong

ACIDIC   NEUTRAL   ALKALINE

Note that:

- pH values below 7 are considered acidic whilst those over 7 are considered as alkaline.
- that an alkaline solution does, in fact, contain hydrogen ions. The 'neutral' reference point of pH = 7 is that of pure water, which dissociates very weakly into hydrogen and hydroxyl (OH^-) ions, and has a hydrogen ion concentration of 10^{-7} moles/litre ($= 10^{-4}$ millimoles per litre). An alkaline solution contains even fewer hydrogen ions than does water. In acidic solutions, hydrogen ions are in excess of those found in water.
- that increased pH values reflect a decreasing concentration of hydrogen ions, and vice versa.
- that each pH unit change actually represents a ten-fold change in hydrogen ion concentration. For example, a solution at pH of 6 contains 10^{-6} millimoles of hydrogen ions per litre, that is 10× that of water at pH7. This also means that gastric acid with a pH of 3 is just four pH units lower than that of water but it has 10^{-3} millimoles of hydrogen ions per litre, 10,000× that of water!

In view of the reactivity of hydrogen ions, it should not be surprising to find that their concentration in body fluids is maintained at low values. The pH of blood plasma is actually slightly alkaline with a pH of about 7.4. This corresponds to a concentration of 40 nanomoles of hydrogen ions per litre ($= 4 \times 10^{-5}$ millimoles per litre). To put this into the context of extracellular fluid composition generally, this is of the order of 100,000 times less than the concentration of potassium ions ($=$ approximately 4 millimoles per litre) and 3.5 million times less than that of sodium ions ($=$ approximately 140 millimoles per litre); an extremely low concentration indeed.

EXERCISE

What is the concentration of hydrogen ions in stomach acid at a pH of 3?

Buffers

With reference to equation 3.2, the point is made that hydrochloric acid molecules produced when hydrogen ions and chloride ions recombine will instantly

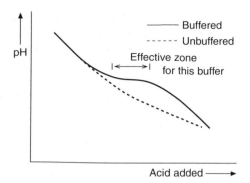

Figure 3.4 **Buffering**
Acidity is associated with low pH values and so in adding acid to a solution, the pH tends to decrease. A buffer acts to maintain a near constancy of pH within its reflective zone by removing free hydrogen ions

Q. Why does the acidity of the solution eventually begin to increase once more?

dissociate again. This means that if we were to add further hydrogen ions to the solution, the excess hydrogen ions would now favour recombination to the acid, but the acid would immediately dissociate. Adding hydrogen ions to the solution therefore would increase its acidity in direct relation to the amount of hydrogen ions added.

In equation 3.3, however, it was noted that a characteristic of a weak acid is that it dissociates poorly. In that example, if further hydrogen ions were added to the solution, many of them would combine with the bicarbonate ions present and form undissociated molecules of carbonic acid. Consequently, few of the added hydrogen ions will remain in solution, thus its acidity will change only slightly (Figure 3.4). This effect is referred to as 'buffering'. Bicarbonate ions, phosphate ions and proteins (e.g. haemoglobin) in blood are important buffers in body fluids, and they act to ensure that hydrogen ion concentration remains very low inside and outside cells.

Physiological actions of electrolytes

It was noted earlier that:

- the exchange of fluid and solute that occurs between blood capillaries and tissue fluid results in an almost identical ionic composition of plasma and tissue fluid (see Table 3.1) and so blood analysis data are taken to be representative of the entire compartment (though not of the transcellular fluids).
- the intracellular fluid has a composition that is very different to the extracellular fluid (Table 3.1). The role of the cell membrane in enabling these differences was explained earlier, but will only be effective if the composition of the tissue fluid that bathes the cells is also regulated.

Although there are quantitative differences between the electrolytes found in the intra- and extracellular fluids, the types of electrolyte present are similar. The following considers some of the actions of the main ionic constituents of body fluids, but also identifies how disturbances are detected.

Sodium (Na$^+$) and chloride (Cl$^-$)

Compared with extracellular fluid, the intracellular fluids contain much lower concentrations of sodium but much higher concentrations of potassium (Table 3.1). This difference is achieved by the activities of a sodium/potassium exchange carrier within the cell membrane of (probably all) cells. The carrier 'pumps' sodium ions out of the cell, and potassium ions into it, and helps to establish an electrical difference between the inner and outer surfaces of the membrane (see Box 3.4).

Box 3.4   Application: differences in the electrical potential across cell membranes

The exchange of sodium and potassium produced by the sodium/potassium pump in cell membranes helps to compensate for a slow diffusional 'leak' of ions across the cell membrane. The concentration gradients for the ions means that sodium tends to diffuse into the cell, and potassium out of it. The potassium (K$^+$) leak is faster than that of sodium and this is actually very useful because, in effect, it means that cells are constantly leaking electrical (positive) charge faster than they gain it (from sodium; Na$^+$), and so produce a voltage difference across a cell membrane. This electrical difference is referred to as a 'resting membrane potential' and is of the order of 70 millivolts (since it is positive charge that leaks out of the cell, in relative terms this means that the inside is more negative than the outside). Note the units; a millivolt is 1/1000 of a volt. The 1.5 volts of a standard AA size battery is massive in comparison! Nevertheless, this membrane potential is crucial in physiological functioning.

Stimulation of nerve or muscle cells causes the cell membrane to become permeable to sodium ions (Figure 3.5), which enter so rapidly down the pronounced diffusional and electrical gradient established by the sodium/potassium pump that the membrane 'depolarizes' and becomes positive inside. This change in the polarity of the membrane potential is called an 'action potential'. Restoration of the resting state necessitates removing this excess positive charge and is achieved by the membrane becoming very permeable to potassium ions, which rapidly diffuse out of the cell down their concentration gradient. The lost potassium ions (and accumulated sodium ions) are re-exchanged by the sodium/potassium pump, thus preventing a cumulative disturbance in intracellular ion concentrations. Once the action potential is finished, the ionic permeabilities reset at the basal values and so the resting potential is restored. Action potentials are used to produce nerve impulses, and to activate muscle contraction.

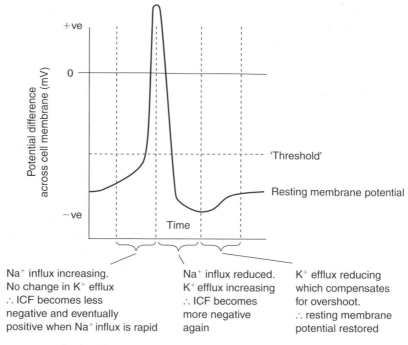

Na⁺ influx increasing.
No change in K⁺ efflux
∴ ICF becomes less
negative and eventually
positive when Na⁺ influx is rapid

Na⁺ influx reduced.
K⁺ efflux increasing
∴ ICF becomes
more negative
again

K⁺ efflux reducing
which compensates
for overshoot.
∴ resting membrane
potential restored

Figure 3.5 **Roles of sodium and potassium ions in generating an action potential in a nerve cell**
Notice how the voltage (potential difference) across the cell membrane is changed by the movement of sodium or potassium ions (i.e. movement of positive charge)

Q. Why is the first phase of the action potential (when sodium ions enter the cell) referred to as a depolarization?

EXERCISE

Refer to Chapter 8 and identify how local anaesthetics influence the sodium/potassium exchange pumps in cell membranes to prevent the passage of action potentials along a nerve fibre.

Sodium ions also influence other cell membrane processes. For example, the sodium concentration gradient across the membrane facilitates the carriage of substances such as glucose and amino acids into cells by a process called 'facilitated diffusion'.

Chloride ions have less widespread effects than sodium. In particular, they may interfere with the electrical properties of cell membranes in parts of the central nervous system. They can do this because they are negatively charged, and are present in relatively large concentrations in extracellular fluid. Thus, a change in the permeability of the membrane to these ions will allow a rapid diffusion of chloride into the cell. The negative charge carried by these ions acts to increase the polarization of the resting membrane (i.e. the negativity of the inside of the cell membrane is increased; see Box 3.4). This makes the membrane potential less likely to reach the threshold value (see Figure 3.5) that admits sodium during an action potential. In effect, this inhibits the nerve cell and prevents its stimulation.

The concentration of sodium and chloride ions within plasma must therefore be regulated. Their abundance in extracellular fluid means that they are the major ionic determinant of its osmotic potential (see Box 3.1) and so an increase in their concentration will cause water to move out of cells by osmosis. Conversely, should their extracellular concentration fall, then the osmotic potential is decreased and water enters cells. In other words, the changes produce characteristics observed during dehydration or overhydration. Responses to change the excretion of water would be appropriate (described in Box 3.6) but, in addition, they must also stimulate the excretion of sodium chloride. Sodium chloride content and water balance are therefore inextricably linked, and the detection of a change in sodium chloride content entails stretch receptors within the venous circulation and right side of the heart which monitor the volume of blood.

Potassium (K$^+$)

The concentration gradient for potassium across cell membranes also affects the electrical potential of the membrane (Table 3.1 and Box 3.4). An increase in extracellular potassium concentration would reduce the concentration gradient and so interfere with the rate of diffusion of potassium out of the cell. This in turn would make the electrical difference begin to approach the threshold at which nerve and muscle cells are activated (see Figure 3.5), and so these tissues would become more excitable. If the concentration continues to rise, however, the membrane's electrical properties will be unable to return to the normal resting state and so the cell becomes incapable of being stimulated. Thus, if one monitored heart rate, it might increase as the extracellular potassium concentration rises, becomes dysrhythmic (observed as an abnormal EDG recording, and a loss of normal sinus rhythm) and would eventually cease.

Similarly, a decrease in extracellular potassium concentration causes the diffusional 'leak' of potassium to increase and the membrane potential to deviate away from the threshold, thus making the cell more difficult, perhaps even impossible, to stimulate. Once again, if we were monitoring heart rate then it would decrease as potassium concentration diminished.

The regulation of plasma potassium concentration is therefore vital; it is monitored directly by specialized receptor cells within the adrenal gland.

EXERCISE

What is the homeostatic range for potassium concentration in plasma? Why is it so narrow?

Calcium (Ca^{2+})

The calcium ion concentration in extracellular fluid is low compared with that of sodium and potassium. The concentration actually represents only about half of the total calcium present since some calcium is found bound to plasma proteins. Many calcium salts, for example calcium phosphate, have a low solubility in water. The concentration of calcium ions in extracellular fluid is close to that at which such salts will start to precipitate out and form deposits within blood vessels (= arteriosclerosis) and so both calcium and phosphate concentrations must be kept quite low. Calcium ions in the extracellular fluid also influence the threshold membrane potential at which excitable cells are stimulated (see Figure 3.5). A reduction in calcium ion concentration reduces the threshold and makes the cells more easily stimulated and hence more excitable. This could cause powerful muscle spasms, called tetany. If calcium ion concentration is increased, nerve and muscle cells become less excitable and so the cells become more difficult to stimulate (for example, bowel contractions may slow or even cease). The need to regulate the extracellular calcium concentration is clear; the concentration is monitored directly by cells within the thyroid and parathyroid glands.

Calcium ions have roles in various processes within cells, for example in mediating muscle contraction. Their concentration in cells is actually quite low but more is bound to protein; thus, the availability of calcium ions may be increased rapidly as required. By controlling calcium availability, cells are therefore able to regulate calcium-dependent processes.

Hydrogen (H$^+$), bicarbonate (HCO$_3^-$) and phosphate (PO$_4^{2-}$)

Hydrogen ions are a product of normal metabolic reactions. Their low concentration in extracellular fluid arises partly because they are 'buffered' (see Figure 3.4 and p. 68 and earlier discussion) and partly because they are excreted efficiently in urine (their carbon dioxide source is also efficiently excreted). The reactivity of hydrogen ions is such that their concentration must be kept very low, but not so low as to produce an alkalosis (see Box 3.5). The receptors involved are respiratory chemoreceptors (peripheral receptors; see Chapter 6) and kidney cells.

Bicarbonate ions are abundant in extracellular fluid and are important 'buffers' of hydrogen ions. Phosphate ions are more important in this respect inside cells (their concentration in extracellular fluid must be kept low; see 'Calcium' above). The bicarbonate concentration of blood plasma may be altered by changes to renal excretion of the ion in response to acidity changes.

Phosphate ions within cells are also an integral part of metabolic processes. For example, compounds such as adenosine triphosphate (ATP) act as energy-carriers that make the energy released from metabolic fuels available to chemical processes within the cell (Chapter 6).

Box 3.5   Application: acidosis and alkalosis

'Acidosis' is defined by a group of signs and symptoms (headache, blurred vision, fatigue, weakness, possibly tremors and delirium) arising from an excess of hydrogen ions in body fluids, which makes them more acidic (i.e. a pH value less than 7.35). It is usually as a consequence of:

- carbon dioxide retention. As noted in the text, carbon dioxide combines with water to form carbonic acid. The role of this respiratory gas in promoting the acidosis is recognized by referring to this as 'respiratory acidosis'.
- excessive metabolic acid production. This is referred to as 'metabolic acidosis' but the precise acid that is generated depends upon the cause; for example, ketoacidosis in diabetes mellitus, lactic acidosis in strenuous exercise.
- inadequate excretion of hydrogen ions, for example in renal failure. This, too, is usually referred to as a metabolic acidosis.

Similarly, alkalosis is defined by a group of signs and symptoms (weakness, muscle cramps, dizziness, carpopedal spasm, paresthesia) arising from insufficient hydrogen ions in body fluids, thus making them more alkaline than they should be (i.e. a pH value greater than 7.45). This is usually as a consequence of:

- inadequate generation of acids (in this the syndrome is referred to as either a respiratory or metabolic alkalosis), or
- excessive presence of buffer chemicals that act to lower the acidity.

EXERCISE

Using a textbook, identify the roles of the following hormones in regulating body fluid volume and composition:

- antidiuretic hormone.
- aldosterone.
- angiotensin II.
- calcitonin.
- parathyroid hormone.
- atrial natriuretic factor.

Perioperative influences on water and electrolyte homeostasis

Provided that water and electrolytes are distributed normally within the body, the body fluids will remain in a steady state if additions of water or electrolytes are matched with losses. Therefore, there must be a balance between water and salts entering the fluids through our diets or through synthesis by metabolism, and through losses from the body by excretory processes or otherwise. A schema for water and electrolyte homeostasis is shown in Figure 3.6.

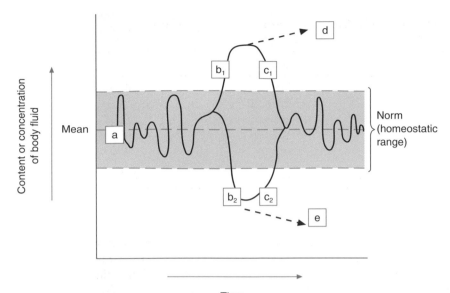

Figure 3.6 Body fluid homeostasis

a   Body fluid composition varying but remaining within the homeostatic range (i.e. fluid composition is optimal)

b   Body fluid composition outside the homeostatic range, e.g. excessive body fluid volume b_1, or dehydration b_2

c_1, c_1 Return of body fluid composition to within homeostatic range, by physiological processes

d, e   Persistent disturbance of body fluid composition, perhaps as a consequence of illness or surgery. Inadequacy of physiological responses will make intervention necessary if body fluid composition is to be normalized.

Source: adapted from Clancy, J. and McVicar, A.J. (2002) *Physiology and Anatomy: a Homeostatic Approach, Second Edition.* London: Arnold.

Q. Can you use this graph to explain how the body responds to being overhydrated?

Water balance

The water that is added to body fluids is drunk, is in our food (even the driest of cereals contains some water), and is generated in cells as a product of respiration reactions (Table 3.2). In the UK, the cool climate means that most of the time water will largely be lost from the body in urine, though sweat can become the main route during hot weather as evaporation is used to promote heat loss from the body.

Water lost via evaporation from the airways and sweat is referred to as 'insensible' water loss because the saturation of respiratory gases with water vapour is

Table 3.2 Water balance. Figures shown are 'typical' for a temperate (i.e. UK) climate

Water input (ml per day)		Water output (ml per day)	
Drink	1500	Urine	1400
Food	800	Evaporation	
Metabolic production	200	Lungs	500
		Skin	400
		Faeces	200
Total	**2500**	**Total**	**2500**

unavoidable and sweat production relates to our need to maintain temperature homeostasis, irrespective of our state of hydration. This means that water balance is mainly controlled by changing intake (of drinking water) and by regulating the urinary or faecal losses. These latter are adjusted according to our state of hydration and so are referred to as 'sensible' losses. Faecal losses, however, are relatively less important in this respect than urinary ones. Nevertheless, dehydration is a common cause of constipation.

Controlling urine production therefore is essential in the maintenance of hydration. When we are overhydrated, we must produce large volumes of dilute urine, so dilute that water is lost from the body more efficiently than solutes, thus raising the osmotic potential of body fluids. If we are dehydrated we must produce low volumes of urine that is more concentrated than body fluids, so that water is conserved more efficiently than solutes and the osmotic potential of body fluids will decrease.

The switch from producing a high volume, dilute urine to a low volume, concentrated one is produced by antidiuretic hormone (ADH; anti- = against, diuretic = promote urination) which enhances the water permeability of the collecting ducts of the kidneys. Central to the determination of urine concentration and volume, then, is the degree to which ADH is released from the posterior pituitary gland. This depends upon the osmotic potential (i.e. level of hydration) of the plasma and how much it has deviated from its homeostatic set-point of about 285 milliosmole/l. Any change in plasma osmotic potential outside its homeostatic range is detected by specialized nerve cells, called osmoreceptors, within the hypothalamus.

The mechanism of ADH release is very sensitive, but it is important to note that our need to excrete urea and electrolytes means that we must produce some urine, even if we are dehydrated. Zero urine production (and water loss) is not an option in health. The availability of drinking water is therefore essential for survival. Provided that water is available to drink, our water balance is maintained within the limits of ±2 per cent of the homeostatic set-point. The response is relatively quick. For example, drinking a litre of water results in the excretion of any excess within one to two hours.

Pre-operative influences on water balance

The risk of respiratory failure arising as a consequence of gastric aspiration (see Box 6.6; Chapter 6), is reduced by restricting food and water intake for a period prior to the surgery. The minimum length of that period has been debated for many years: in a seminal piece of work, Hamilton-Smith (1972) reported how hospital policies varied and how fasting times were based on routine and tradition. Sadly, little seems to have changed in the interim period, and fasting periods ranging from a few hours to more than a day have been reported; eleven hours seems to be about the median period (Chapman 1996; Jester and Williams 1999; Rowe 2000).

Reasonable pre-operative periods of restriction (i.e. 'nil by mouth') should not induce a major water imbalance, but long periods will mean that patients entering the operating theatre are already dehydrated. Studies have demonstrated that a positive fluid balance prior to surgery can actually improve outcomes (Garrison *et al.* 1996) and pre-operative fasting is an issue that warrants further work. Based on gastric emptying times, some authors have advocated a pre-operative period of food fasting of four to six hours, and an even shorter period of two to four hours for fluid restriction (Chapman 1996; Soreide *et al.* 1996; Corbett and Mortimer 1997).

Age and any underlying medical conditions are additional pre-operative (indeed, perioperative) influences on fluid balance in surgical patients. Fluid homeostasis is less efficient in older people and in very young children, and this makes these groups particularly susceptible to dehydration. Other factors such as pyrexia, diuretic use, enemata or vomiting will also have potential consequences for fluid balance status. Where possible, any imbalance should be reduced prior to surgery.

EXERCISE

Identify the pre-operative fasting regime in your clinical area, and the rationale for its duration.

Intra-operative and post-operative influences on water balance

The effects of surgery on fluid balance will vary depending upon the type of surgery, the time taken and the skills of the surgical team. This section can only provide an outline of the process and will consider only the potential for fluid disturbance, primarily in relation to major surgery. Some factors will relate to both the intra- and post-operative periods and it is logical to consider an overview of factors from both.

The output side of the balance 'equation' in Table 3.2 is markedly altered by surgery.

■ Urinary output may be decreased because of dehydration, because of depressed renal function (even acute renal failure) arising from the effects of surgery, or because of the prevailing hormonal background (see below,

p. 79). Depressed renal function after major surgery is not unusual, leading to inadequate urine production (oliguria) or even an absence of urine production (anuria) (see Box 3.6). Conversely, urine volume may even be very large post-operatively because of a 'rebound' in kidney function following a period of reduced perfusion during surgery.

- Faecal losses may be increased in the post-operative period through the onset of diarrhoea (see p. 84).

- Respiratory losses might be enhanced because of ventilation procedures or because of anxiety or pain in the post-operative period.

- Sweat losses will increase post-operatively if there is infection or if there is pain. Also, a humid hospital environment or excessive bedclothes encourages these 'insensible' losses because temperature homeostasis is difficult if sweat cannot evaporate; thus more sweat is produced.

Box 3.6   Application: acute renal failure

Acute renal failure is frequently observed if the kidneys have received poor supplies of blood, for example in some lengthy surgical procedures, or following severe haemorrhage (Stewart and Barnett 1997; Seaton-Mills 1999). Acute renal failure caused by poor blood supply is referred to as having a *pre-renal* cause. It may be several hours or even several days after clinical intervention before the kidneys resume normal filtration. The failure may also have a *renal* or *post-renal* cause. The latter commonly occurs if there is ureteral, or urethral, obstruction, leading to back-pressure of retained urine on the kidneys. Renal causes are not fully understood, but usually involve *acute tubular necrosis* (ATN), a disruption of nephron structure possibly produced by infections or toxic chemicals. In this instance, recovery may take several months. The reasons for the delay in recovery from acute renal failure remain unclear, and in some people function may never be completely restored.

Acute renal failure (ARF) is a condition characterized by a sudden, rapid deterioration in glomerular filtration ratio (GFR) and renal function.

- Oliguria is observed (i.e. less than 30 ml urine/hour or less than 400 ml in 24 hours). In some instances renal function can be so depressed as to cause anuria (0–100 ml urine/24 hours). The lower limit for 'normal' function relates to the ability of kidneys to conserve water when we are dehydrated. Thus urine production may be very low, but the urine will not be as concentrated as would be anticipated had the patient been very dehydrated. Also, the patient's appearance would not indicate dehydration of this magnitude.

- Uraemia is present – a raised blood urea concentration. Urea (and uric acid) are especially dependent upon an adequate GFR for their excretion. Uraemia (and uricaemia) is often indicative of an inability to excrete the normal load. The uraemia may cause blood clotting irregularities.

■ Potassium concentration is elevated in blood plasma. In the absence of a potassium infusion, hyperkalaemia is almost certainly due to an inability to excrete potassium normally. Failure to maintain electrolyte balance may lead to raised serum potassium sufficient to cause fatal cardiac arrhythmias; this is often the cause of death in ARF.

■ An acidosis is present. The acidosis is of a cellular or 'metabolic' origin and arises as a consequence of a failure to excrete hydrogen ions. Acidosis causes the rate and depth of breathing to be slightly elevated.

■ The numbers of white cells in a blood sample are often increased in ATN (acute tubular necrosis, one of the causes of ARF) where there is infection or toxins present.

Additional imbalances produced by the renal dysfunction will be:

■ fluid overload. This is partly due to water retention and partly due to an expansion of the extracellular fluid compartment as a consequence of sodium retention. Peripheral oedema might be observed. In severe cases pulmonary oedema may occur.

■ poor appetite, nausea and vomiting arising from the disturbed blood composition.

■ changes in mentation such as drowsiness and confusion, again as a consequence of altered blood composition.

The specific goal of care for someone in acute renal failure is to try to normalize, as far as possible, the body fluid composition by managing dietary input. In this way a new homeostatic balance can be established so that input once again equals output.

ARF usually has three phases:

1 the oliguric phase.
2 the diuretic phase. This phase can follow after several days, several weeks, or even several months (in ATN) and is usually indicative that the kidneys are recovering.
3 The recovery phase. The diuresis declines and homeostasis is re-established without the need for restricted dietary inputs.

Body fluid management may still be required even when the diuretic phase commences because the kidneys are initially unable to concentrate the urine. Strict monitoring therefore is essential throughout the course of ARF.

In addition to influencing these usual routes of water loss, surgery also introduces additional routes of potentially significant loss. These are identified in Table 3.3; dehydration from exposed tissues is likely to be the main concern.

Table 3.3 Additional sources of water loss in the perioperative period

Source	Comment
Evaporation	Occurs when moist tissues are exposed to the atmosphere. Measures are taken during surgery to reduce it but losses can still be extensive.
Blood loss	Unavoidable, though minimized.
Wound drains	Tissue fluid produced as inflammatory exudate. Normally removed by drainage to facilitate wound healing.
Loss of peritoneal fluid	Fluid loss from the abdominal cavity is unavoidable in laparotomy.
Vomiting or nasogastric aspirate	Loss of ingested water, and gastric secretions.

Note
Loss of tissue fluid if a patient has burns will be another major factor.

EXERCISE

Distinguish between 'sensible' and 'insensible' water losses.

Of further consideration is the effect of surgery on the endocrine system. Surgery is a trauma, albeit one that is controlled, and injury stimulates the release of various hormones (Chapter 7). The following promote water (and sodium) conservation:

■ *adrenaline* (and sympathetic nerve activity associated with it). Adrenaline (or *epinephrine* as it is known in the USA) is released in response to surgical stress and blood loss. It has direct and indirect actions to enhance sodium and water conservation by the kidneys.
■ *aldosterone*. The adrenaline/sympathetic nerve response to surgery will stimulate the release of renin from the kidneys. This in turn promotes formation of angiotensin II (a potent vasoconstrictor) that also stimulates the release of aldosterone from the adrenal cortex. This hormone promotes sodium and water retention by the kidneys (and potassium excretion).
■ *antidiuretic hormone* (ADH or vasopressin). This hormone will be released as a consequence of anaesthesia-induced hypotension, blood loss, because there has been physical contact with/manipulation of internal organs, or because of dehydration. The vasoconstrictor actions of this hormone help to maintain blood pressure, and its actions on the kidneys promotes water conservation.

Implications for managing water balance

The loss of water from the body during and after surgery is subject to many influencing factors, some of which promote increased water loss, and some water retention. The exact net effect is too difficult to quantify in practice, but generally an overall loss of water might be anticipated in major surgery and patients will usually be dehydrated to some degree. Rehydration over twenty-four hours is ideal but the possible continued release of the hormones identified above, especially if the patient is in pain and/or distressed, should be considered when assessing fluid balance status.

Assessment is very important here.

- A reduced haemoglobin concentration of blood, depressed renal function and reduced central venous pressure (if measured) are all indicators of reduced blood volume.
- Assessment of the volumes of tissue fluid and intracellular compartments are difficult and not normally performed in practice. Assessing fluid balance status may be done by repeated weighing of the patient, but this is a very crude indicator.
- Constructing fluid balance charts is therefore fundamental to many areas of nursing practice. Volumes of fluid consumed or infused can be matched with readily measured outputs of urine, of wound drains and, if applicable, of nasogastric aspirates. Other routes, such as vomiting, diarrhoea and evaporative losses are more difficult to assess. Again, fluid balance charts may only be crude indicators.

The dietary input of water is obviously not going to be a consideration during surgery but is a factor in the post-operative period (and pre-operatively, see above, p. 76). Of more importance to this discussion is the use of infusions to restore hydration. The type of infusate will vary, depending upon the losses likely to have been sustained during the procedure (see 'Infusates and the support of body fluid compartments', p. 85).

Referring to Table 3.2, it can be seen that an input of about 2.5 litres of water per day is normally required (in a UK climate). In the clinical setting it is more usual to aim for 3 litres per day to compensate for additional losses, but this rate of fluid administration will only be appropriate if renal function is normal and there are no underlying complications. In reality, normal urine output is unlikely in the initial 24–48 hours after major surgery because of intra-operative dehydration, or because of the retentive influences of hormones, or even because of depressed renal function. Difficulty in establishing the actual physiological status of the patient means that care must be exercised to ensure that the individual does not swing from a situation of dehydration to one of overhydration.

The intake of fluid should not exceed the measured output by more than 1 litre per 24 hours (i.e. a volume to compensate for unmeasured 'insensible' losses; Table 3.2). This assumes that renal function relates only to the hydration status

Table 3.4 Signs of altered water balance

Dehydration	• Dry mouth, may reflect the lack of oral fluids or mouth breathing, but could indicate a significant change in water balance. • Reduced skin turgor. See Box 3.3. • If the patient can communicate, then complaining of a headache, or the exhibiting of behavioural/attitude change may also be indicators of dehydration.
Overhydration	• Hypervolaemia producing dyspnoea, increased central venous pressure (distended neck veins), oedema. • Loss of appetite. • Headache. • Behavioural disturbance, apprehension, agitation.

of the individual and that evaporative losses are average or only slightly elevated. As noted earlier, renal function may be depressed in the post-operative period because blood flow to the kidneys was disrupted during the operation. Thus, a low urine volume could be indicative of either dehydration or depressed renal function (see Box 3.7); depressed renal function will continue to cause fluid retention even if hydration returns to normal.

Therefore the situation post-operatively is one in which a patient is likely initially to be fluid retentive. If a patient is dependent upon infusions for the majority of fluid intake, the complications introduced by surgery make it difficult to 'guesstimate' the most appropriate rate of fluid delivery. It is not unusual for the type of infusate, and its rate of administration, to be standardized according to the type of surgery performed, and so it is important that fluid balance charts are supplemented with other observations to reduce the risk of prolonging dehydration, or to avoid excessive overhydration. Indicators for this are identified in Table 3.4.

Box 3.7   Application: low urine volume

Urine production in health may be as low as 30 ml per hour, equivalent to about 700 ml per day. The production of such small volumes would be indicative of severe dehydration and so the urine has a characteristic dark yellow colour and is very concentrated. Urine production in the post-operative period that is lower than 30 ml/hour usually indicates depressed renal function, provided that urinary retention in the bladder is not occurring. The urine will also be lighter in colour and less concentrated than might be anticipated for such an apparent degree of dehydration.

Even with a moderate renal output, the possibility of diminished glomerular filtration rate cannot be excluded. A diminished glomerular filtration rate might be confirmed by observing blood urea and creatinine concentrations. The efficient excretion of these substances depends upon an adequate rate of glomerular filtration, as the influence of renal tubular functioning on urea excretion in urine formation is not as pronounced as for other urinary constituents, and for creatinine is virtually zero. Poor filtration will result in urea and creatinine concentrations in blood rising above normal. Under such circumstances, urinary output of water and electrolytes may be encouraged by the use of diuretic drugs, but this must be balanced with a modified input.

EXERCISE

When is urine volume considered to be so low as to be of concern?

Electrolyte balance

Most of the electrolytes that are ingested in our foods are absorbed. The most prevalent ones in our diets are sodium, potassium and chloride. Although abundant in body fluids, these ions are not stored to any degree by the body and their balance is determined by adjusting their output from the body, mainly in the urine, so that it matches the input. A sodium balance chart is depicted in Table 3.5: the role of kidney function in the regulation of sodium balance is clear. Sodium excretion is regulated by a number of hormones that are released according to the volume status of the extracellular fluid, especially angiotensin, aldosterone and atrial natriuretic factor.

Calcium balance is complicated by the presence of substantial stores of this mineral within bone and so maintaining a balance entails controlling uptake from the bowel, uptake/release from bone, and urinary excretion. Only about 50 per cent of dietary intake is normally absorbed from the bowel, depending upon the state of calcium balance and of the dietary calcium content. If the individual is deficient then the proportion may be increased, but the ion will also be released from 'stores' in bone, in order to restore the plasma calcium concentration. This helps to reduce the short-term impact of any deficit.

Some electrolytes, such as hydrogen ions and bicarbonate ions, are also produced through metabolic processes. Their excretion must also match this additional source, as well as any dietary intake. It was noted earlier that the concentration of hydrogen ions may also be 'buffered' by bicarbonate ions.

Table 3.5 Sodium balance. Figures are representative for a 'normal' diet in the UK

Sodium input	mmole/day	Sodium output	mmole/day
Food	180	Urine	160
		Faeces/sweat	20
Total	180 (approx = 8 g)	Total	180 (approx = 8 g)

Some of the extra fluid that is lost during surgery, for example in wound drains, produces a combined water and electrolyte deficit, and so may have little effect on the net concentration of the electrolytes in plasma. In addition, there is so much potassium within cells, and calcium in bone, that their secretion into extracellular fluid means that a persistently decreased plasma concentration of these ions may not necessarily be observed even though the individual is in deficit. The use of blood samples to monitor electrolyte balance is therefore limited, although any changes in composition that are observed will clearly suggest a disturbance has occurred.

However, an electrolyte imbalance is likely and will be exacerbated if there is vomiting and/or diarrhoea. Whilst infusions may prevent electrolyte changes, or restore them to normality, the difficulties in assessing a deficit, and the possibility of resultant overload, means that patients should be observed for changes in electrolyte composition. This is particularly important for sodium (chloride) because of its relationship with extracellular fluid volume (and hence blood volume), potassium and calcium as these influence the excitable cells of the body, that is, nerve and muscle cells, and hydrogen ions (i.e. blood pH).

Perioperative influences on electrolyte balance: vomiting

Vomiting is a potentially serious problem because of the risk of aspiration into the airways, possibly causing pneumonia if the aspirate is inhaled into the alveoli (see Chapter 6). Also, vomitus contains an abundance of sodium, chloride and potassium ions, but is also very acidic because of the presence of gastric acid. Loss of gastric fluid by vomiting simply means that the stomach secretes more and persistent loss of gastric fluid may induce a serious loss of electrolytes (and water), including hydrogen ions. A metabolic alkalosis may ensue.

Vomiting (or emesis) is co-ordinated by the vomiting (or emetic) centre in the medulla oblongata; stimulation of the vomiting centre occurs at the chemoreceptor trigger zone. This area is not protected by the blood–brain barrier and so may be stimulated by blood-borne drugs and toxins. Signals from the vomiting centre pass to the vagus nerve (a parasympathetic nerve) and to the spinal motor neurons which supply the abdominal muscles and so initiate the vomiting response. Peristaltic contraction of the bowel is reversed causing the contents of the upper intestine to move into the stomach. The glottis closes, and breath holding and relaxation of the oesophagus and gastric sphincter occur. When the abdominal muscles contract the gastric contents are ejected.

EXERCISE
What is meant by the term 'blood–brain barrier'?

Vomiting may occur at almost any time during the perioperative phase. The only time it will not occur is when the patient is paralysed by neuromuscular blocking agents, and under deep anaesthesia (Carrie *et al.* 1997). Anaesthetic drugs can induce nausea and vomiting, as can opioid analgesics (Neal 1997; Griffiths 2000), therefore the homeostatic control for prevention is through anti-emetic drug therapy and pre-operative precautions such as fasting and specialist bowel preparations in cases involving surgery on the gastrointestinal tract. Treatment with anti-emetics should be given before any emetic stimulus occurs and can be given with premedication, on induction of anaesthesia or intravenously during anaesthesia (Neal 1997).

Drugs such as metoclopramide have an anti-nausea and anti-emetic effect; it is a dopamine antagonist and blocks the central dopamine receptors in the chemoreceptor trigger zone. There is also an increase in stomach contractions and enhanced tone of the lower oesophageal sphincter which speed normal gastric emptying and absorption of other drugs such as analgesics, which in turn produces an enhanced analgesic effect. Domperidone acts in a similar way to metoclopramide.

Newer anti-emetic drugs with fewer side effects are now being used in conjunction with general anaesthesia. Ondansetron is a serotonin (5-HT$_3$) antagonist; there are 5-HT$_3$ receptors within the chemoreceptor trigger zone and gut, and it is thought that these receptors activate the vagal sensory fibres to the vomiting centre that lead to reflex nausea and vomiting. Ondansetron has fewer side effects than the dopamine antagonists although it can cause constipation and headaches (Neal 1997).

The control of nausea and vomiting during the perioperative phase is not solely reliant upon the use of anti-emetic drug therapy. As stated above, vomiting can occur at any time except when the patient is under deep anaesthesia, so it is essential that at any other time every precaution is taken to avoid vomiting.

EXERCISE

Readers interested in the pharmacology of controlling vomiting might find it useful to read pages 162–74 and 219–23 in Carrie et al. (1997).

Perioperative influences on electrolyte balance: post-operative diarrhoea

Diarrhoea is common following surgery to the gastrointestinal tract. Patients who require surgery for diseases of their intestinal tract often present pre-operatively with symptoms that include diarrhoea. Prior to surgery, most patients will have a bowel preparation in order to empty the bowel of faeces. This preparation can cause profuse diarrhoea in the pre-operative phase. However, this is also necessary to reduce the possibility of faecal contamination of the surgical field and at the site of bowel anastomosis. When large sections of the bowel have been removed there may be severe diarrhoea post-operatively (Forrest et al. 1995) as this compromises the absorption of fluid by the bowel.

Anti-emetic drugs such as metoclopramide and domperidone (see above) also act as motility stimulants, speeding the transit of the contents from the stomach and causing contractions in the intestine. Therefore, it is possible that patients undergoing other types of surgery may also experience some post-operative diarrhoea if given these drugs.

It is important that the faecal output is monitored closely as fluid and electrolyte loss can be substantial. This is because the bowel secretes several litres of fluid per day, primarily into the stomach and duodenum, and little of this will be reabsorbed again in someone who has diarrhoea. Secretion will continue, leading to potentially severe loss of fluid. The fluid will contain electrolytes, especially bicarbonate ions (the pancreas secretes an alkaline, bicarbonate-rich fluid). Persistent diarrhoea therefore will promote a severe electrolyte loss and a metabolic acidosis.

Fluid replacement therapy and parenteral nutrition may be necessary. Codeine phosphate therapy may be necessary to combat the diarrhoea and antisecretory drugs, e.g. Ranitidine, are used to reduce gastric hypersecretion. Infection and skin breakdown around a stoma site, the wound and the anus can also rapidly develop as a result of the altered nutritional state. Nutrient replacement therapy is therefore essential.

Infusates and the support of body fluid compartments

A variety of fluids, such as saline or dextrose, may be infused intravenously to support the volume and/or composition of body fluid compartments. Blood products may also be infused but, plasma and plasma-products apart, these will also contain cellular components. Nevertheless, such products support the intravascular volume of which plasma is a part and must be considered in relation to body fluid maintenance.

When using plasma protein substitutes and other types of infusate, a distinction may be made according to the solubility of the infusate constituents (see Box 3.1). Accordingly, the infusates used in the perioperative period are considered under three headings: blood products, colloids and crystalloids.

Blood products administered as infusions

Development of technologies in the 1960s and 1970s enabled separation of blood into its components. Whole blood is not now used for infusions because it is more selective to use the individual blood products. Commonly used blood products during surgery are:

- white cell depleted whole blood. White cells are removed to reduce the risk of transmission of infectious agents that may have infected the white cells, such as the prion protein that produces Creutzfeldt-Jakob disease (CJD). It is used when there is life-threatening haemorrhage to rapidly restore the circulating blood volume.
- red cell concentrate. This is commonly used in routine surgery. It replaces red cells lost as a consequence of bleeding.
- fresh frozen plasma. This is often used when patients are having vascular surgery. Anticoagulation is usual in such surgical procedure when blood is diverted away from the site of operation, and externalized. Infusing intact plasma replaces the clotting factors.

> ## Box 3.8   Application: intravenous catheterization
>
> Access to the vascular compartment must be made aseptically to prevent the introduction of infectious agents. The access is normally through:
>
> - peripheral venepuncture in which a needle is inserted through the skin into a superficial vein, often in the hand or arm, and connected to a catheter tubing. The purpose of the intravenous cannula is to facilitate regular blood sampling, to infuse a medication, to commence fluid therapy or to administer radio-opaque/radioactive material.
> - insertion of a large-bore catheter into a major vein, normally a subclavian vein, internal jugular vein or femoral vein. Such catheters enable the measurement of central venous pressure or to deliver large volumes of fluids or viscous fluids as are used in total parenteral nutrition.
>
> Infusates may be administered using a bag/drip feed method in which gravity and blood flow at the needle tip encourage the addition of fluid to blood at the needle tip, or via a pump (syringe driver).
> Complications (see Workman 1999) may arise from:
>
> - phlebitis. This is a redness and swelling of skin at the site of venepuncture. Irritation or pain is usually present. The inflammation represents a defence response to either infection, the chemicals being delivered into the vein, or to the needle/catheter material. Apart from being unpleasant for the patient, phlebitis also raises the risk of blood clotting (= thrombophlebitis) at the needle tip sufficient to cause an embolus.
> - extravasation because the needle tip has exited through the wall of the vein, leading to infusate delivery into the surrounding tissue, resulting in swelling (i.e. oedema) and pallor as blood flow to the area is compromised.
> - blockage, either at the tip of the needle (protein deposition, blood clot, or compression of tissue against it) or through a kink in the catheter tubing.

- platelet concentrate. This is administered to patients who are bleeding following a massive blood transfusion, and helps to restore the capacity to coagulate blood.
- human albumin solution. This is used infrequently, but may be administered if there has been extensive loss of plasma protein, for example in patients with severe burns.

Colloidal infusates: plasma expanders

As the term indicates, plasma expanders provide support for the intravascular volume. They may be protein (for example, Gelofusine; Haemaccel) or carbohydrate (e.g. low or high molecular weight dextrans). Both types are infused as substitutes for plasma proteins and are used as a short-term means of expanding plasma volume, and also to restore the colloid osmotic pressure of plasma and hence the fluid exchange processes across capillary membranes (see earlier, p. 61). Proteinaceous infusates are normally used because they are cleared from the body less rapidly than the dextrans, and dextrans may also induce changes in capillary permeability and thus leak out into tissue fluid. Proteins, though, are more antigenic than dextrans and the recipient must be closely observed for indications of an immune response.

Crystalloid infusates

Box 3.9 Application: isotonic, hypertonic and hypotonic infusates

The suffix '-tonic' in these terms refers to solution 'strength', in particular in relation to their effects on cell volume should cells be suspended in them.

Isotonic (iso- = same) infusates

Despite their different compositions, 'normal' (0.9 per cent) saline, 5 per cent dextrose solution, and Hartmann's solution have the same osmotic effect on the cell membrane. Remember that osmosis relates to a concentration gradient and not upon individual types of solute: these three solutions have the same overall solute concentration and so have the same osmotic properties. The osmotic potential of these solutions is the same as that of the body fluids themselves, and so cells suspended in them will not show a change in their state of hydration (although with dextrose, cell hydration will gradually increase as the glucose is utilized in cellular respiration – see text). Thus, the three solutions noted here are said to be isotonic to body fluids.

Hypertonic (hyper- = excess, above) infusates

These solutions have an osmotic potential that is greater than that of body fluids. Thus, cells suspended in them will shrink as water is lost by osmosis. Such infusates are not as widely used as isotonic ones but do have a value in practice where there is excessive intracellular hydration, or to promote water movement from a transcellular fluid (e.g. the use of mannitol to remove excess cerebrospinal fluid when there is raised intracranial pressure).

Hypotonic (hypo- = less, below) infusates

Hypotonic infusates are rarely used because these infusates have an osmotic potential less than that of body fluids and so cells will take in water by osmosis, resulting in cell swelling, and even lysis. Isotonic 5 per cent dextrose solution provides a means of slowly improving cell hydration and so is a better alternative.

These infusions should support the electrolyte and water balance within the extracellular and/or intracellular fluid compartments. A variety are available; most are isotonic to normal body fluids (see Table 3.6 and Box 3.9).

Saline. Sodium chloride is found predominantly within the extracellular fluid, and so this infusate largely supports that compartment. The most widely used saline is 'normal' or 'isotonic' saline (0.9 per cent sodium chloride solution; i.e. 0.9 g per 100 ml). This has an osmotic potential similar to that of body fluids and so water in the infusion will not move into cells in any quantity. In some circumstances 'hypertonic' saline may be used (e.g. 2.5 per cent sodium chloride solution) to raise the osmotic pressure of extracellular fluids and so cause the withdrawal of water out of cells by osmosis.

Dextrose. This is a solution of glucose. It is usually administered as an isotonic solution (5 per cent; i.e. 5 g per 100 ml) and so might not be expected to promote water movement in or out of cells. However, unlike saline, the glucose will be taken up by cells and utilized, effectively leaving water behind. The loss of solute means that water can now pass into cells by osmosis, thus helping to hydrate the intracellular fluid. The glucose also provides a small amount of energy.

Dextrose/saline. This infusate combines the advantages of both saline and dextrose in that cell hydration is promoted, but the saline component also helps to ensure that some of the infusion remains within the extracellular compartment.

Hartmann's solution. Hartmann's solution provides a more comprehensive support for extracellular fluid than just saline alone. It is sometimes referred to as a 'lactated Ringer' solution. A Ringer solution is one that has an electrolyte composition that closely matches extracellular fluid: Hartmann's solution approximates to human extracellular fluid except that it contains lactate rather than bicarbonate ions. The lactate ions are converted to bicarbonate by the liver and so bicarbonate is added to blood, but it is added at a much slower rate than if it was in the infusate. This helps to reduce the likelihood of bicarbonate overload and a resultant alkalosis. Hartmann's solution is the infusate of choice for perioperative management.

Potassium. Potassium chloride infusion runs the risk of inducing potassium overload if it is administered too quickly, and so this infusate is not widely used in general settings. If it is required, potassium support is usually provided by Hartmann's solution or by potassium in combination with saline or glucose, in which the potassium concentration is close to the normal values for extracellular fluid.

Table 3.6 Composition of crystalloid infusates

	Na^+ mmol l^{-1}	Cl^- mmol l^{-1}	K^+ mmol l^{-1}	Ca^{2+} mmol l^{-1}	Lactate mmol l^{-1}
5% dextrose	0	0	0	0	0
0.9% saline	153	153	0	0	0
Hartmann's solution (Lactated Ringer)	131	111	5	2	29

EXERCISE

Why is it unfeasible to rehydrate someone by infusing them with water? What would be the consequences?

Summary

- Water in the body forms the fluid compartments inside and outside cells but it is more than just a space-filler.
- A continuous exchange between the compartments facilitates regulation of the compartment volumes and also permits the exchange of dissolved substances.
- Body fluid physiology is concerned with maintenance of fluid balance, and with the regulation of the major electrolyte constituents of the body fluids.
- The maintenance of body water is a classic example of homeostasis at work, and is achieved by matching the water output from the systems with that of input.
- Surgery places additional demands on such processes, and introduces additional routes of fluid loss.
- The water-retentive responses to surgery are also influenced by hormonal responses to trauma.
- Promoting the return to a state of balance and maintaining it is important to patient well-being, facilitating recovery.
- Similarly, surgery may induce significant alterations in electrolyte balance, especially if there is vomiting and/or diarrhoea.
- The hydration and electrolyte needs of the surgical patient are difficult to quantify, thus fluid therapies should be used with caution. Whilst a fluid balance chart provides a means of assessing water balance, its interpretation is not straightforward.
- The use of infusions provides clinicians with the means of supporting body fluid compartments when homeostatic mechanisms have failed or are insufficient to meet demands.

Bibliography

Carrie, L.E.S., Simpson, P.J. and Popat, M.T. (1997) *Understanding Anaesthesia, Third Edition*. Oxford: Butterworth Heinemann.

Chapman, A. (1996) Current theory and practice: a study of pre-operative fasting. *Nursing Standard* 10(18): 33–6.

Clancy, J. and McVicar, A. (2002) *Physiology and Anatomy: A Homeostatic Approach, Second Edition*. London: Arnold.

Corbett, A.R. and Mortimer, A.J. (1997) Pre-operative fasting: how long is necessary? *European Journal of Anaesthesiology* 14(6): 555–7.

Forrest, A.P.M., Carter, D.C. and Macleod, I.B. (1995) *Principles and Practice of Surgery. Third Edition*. London: Churchill Livingston.

Garrison, R.N., Wilson, M.A., Matheson, P.J. and Spain, D.A. (1996) Pre-operative saline loading improves outcome after elective non-cardiac surgical procedures. *Annals of Surgery* 62(3): 23–31.

Griffiths, R. (2000) Anaesthetic drugs. *British Journal of Perioperative Nursing* 10(5): 276–9.

Hamilton-Smith, S.H. (1972) *Nil by Mouth?* Royal College of Nursing Report. London.

Hofman, D., Poare, S. and Cherry, G.W. (1998) The use of short-stretch bandaging to control oedema. *Journal of Wound Care* 7(1): 10–12.

Jester, R. and Williams, S. (1999) Pre-operative fasting: putting research into practice. *Nursing Standard* 13(39): 33–5.

Neal, M.J. (1997) *Medical Pharmacology at a Glance, Third Edition*. Oxford: Blackwell Science.

Phillips, S., Daborn, A.K. and Hatch, D.J. (1994) Pre-operative fasting for paediatric anaesthesia. *British Journal of Anaesthesia* 73(4): 529–36.

Rowe, J. (2000) Preoperative fasting: is it time for a change? *Nursing Times* 96(17): 14–15.

Seal, J. (2000) Autologous blood transfusions. *British Journal of Perioperative Nursing* 10(4): 194–8.

Seaton-Mills, D. (1999) Acute renal failure: causes and considerations in the critically ill patient. *Nursing in Critical Care* 4(6): 293–7.

Soreide, E., Hausken, T., Soreide, J.A. and Steen, P.A. (1996) Gastric emptying of a light hospital breakfast. A study using real time ultrasonography. *Acta Anaesthesiologica Scandinavica* 40(5): 549–53.

Stewart, C.L. and Barnett, R. (1997) Acute renal failure in infants, children and adults. *Critical Care Clinics* 13(3): 575–90.

Wilde, M.H. (1997) Long term indwelling catheter care: conceptualising the research base. *Journal of Advanced Nursing* 25(6): 1252–61.

Workman, B. (1999) Peripheral intravenous therapy management. *Nursing Standard* 14(4): 53–62.

Chapter 4

Perioperative influences on immunological homeostasis and wound healing

Introduction: immunological homeostasis

An understanding of immunological homeostasis is important for perioperative practitioners, because the defences of the human body are continually operating to maintain intracellular integrity by waging warfare on harmful environmental agents. These agents are:

- disease-causing organisms called pathogens (e.g. bacteria, viruses). These are sometimes referred to as immunogens.
- pathogen surface receptors called antigens (Figure 4.1, page 95). Antigenic material is usually proteinaceous, stimulating the production of antibodies.
- pathogenic secretions (e.g. bacterial toxins) are also antigenic.
- environmental pollutants (e.g. dust particles) are evident everywhere, even in the ultra-clean operating theatre environment. Ultrafiltration and air conditioning systems help to reduce environmental pollutants.

Box 4.1   Application: hygiene and anti-microbial drugs in the perioperative environment

Long before a patient arrives in the perioperative environment, activities designed to minimize cross-infection are in progress. The first action is for the perioperative practitioner to change into the correct theatre attire. This is necessary to minimize the risks of infection being carried into the department via the practitioner's own clothing and footwear.

The theatre clothing is used for comfort and to prevent the build up of static from man-made fibre, since static attracts dust and microbes present in the air. The wearing of trousers and top is recommended because loose, floppy clothing are possible sources of contamination as perioperative practitioners move about (NATN 1998).

EXERCISE

Revise the protective functions of the skin, briefly discussed in Chapter 2.

Clean, anti-static footwear should be worn within the operating theatre environment, since blood and body fluid splashes on footwear can form an ideal place for microbial colonization. Jewellery is also an area where microbial colonization can occur, so jewellery must not be worn. Exposed hair presents another source of contamination to the perioperative environment and sterile operating field; the hair should be covered with a cap, which can be discarded should it become contaminated or at the end of the shift. Fingernails are also a potential source of microbial contamination; they should, therefore, be kept clean and short. Recent research indicates that nail extensions are a particular hazard.

The perioperative environment should be kept as clean and dust free as possible. Ventilation systems ensure that regular air changes occur, allowing clean air to circulate over the surgical field, while contaminated air is removed from the operating theatre environment. The walls, floor, lights, equipment and surfaces must be kept clean from dust, blood and body fluids. The suction unit should contain a clean disposable bottle for each new case.

All perioperative practitioners must check any sterile instrument trays, packets and equipment, including all disposable sterile items prior to use. The packaging should be intact and dry, any damage to the packaging could cause the item to become unsterile and contaminated with harmful microorganisms. The expiry date must also be checked; if the item has expired it should not be used, as there is no guarantee that the item is still sterile.

The scrub perioperative practitioner must also check all sterile instrumentation for cleanliness; any debris found on an instrument may contain potentially harmful microorganisms, which could be transmitted to another patient if used. In this situation the instruments must be removed and a fresh set of instruments must be used (NATN 1998; Taylor and Campbell 2000).

EXERCISE

Review the methods of sterilization chosen for different equipment used in theatres.

General hand washing for all perioperative practitioners is essential in the prevention of the spread of infection within the perioperative environment. The techniques for scrubbing, gowning and gloving must be adhered to prior to surgical intervention to minimize the risks of contamination within the sterile field. The surgical scrub is a more lengthy procedure than general hand washing and provides effective removal of microorganisms on the skin, prior to the gowning and gloving procedure.

The perioperative practitioner should select an appropriate scrub solution and nail brush, then set the water at a comfortable temperature and steady flow before beginning the surgical scrub. The hands and arms up to the elbows should be washed and rinsed, the nails only should be brushed and rinsed. Practitioners must avoid using the brush on the skin as it can graze the skin leaving it vulnerable to microbes. The process of hand and arm washing and rinsing is repeated twice more. It is important to avoid splashing water on clothes whilst washing hands as this might eventually wet the sterile gown and compromise its effectiveness. Once the scrub has commenced the taps should only be manoeuvred with the elbows to avoid contamination of the hands and arms during the scrub.

The drying of hands is as important as hand washing and must also be performed with great care. A paper towel is used to dry the hands from the fingertips to towards the elbow and should not be brought back towards the fingertips. One towel is used for each hand in accordance with aseptic techniques. The gown should be picked up from the collar end and opened with care to avoid it touching the floor. It should not be shaken unnecessarily and hands are slipped into the arms of the gown carefully. The gown is then tied back by another practitioner to cover the theatre clothes completely. Gloves are put on using the closed glove technique, to avoid contamination (NATN 1998; Pinney 2000).

EXERCISE

Review the following aseptic techniques used in practice:

- hand washing technique,
- closed glove technique,
- gowning technique,
- opening of sterile packs.

In summary, all activities are related to keeping the patient safe by preventing infection and contamination, to avoid complications for the patient during the post-operative period.

Patients undergoing surgical procedures who are elderly and unwell are more susceptible to colonization by pathogenic organisms and subsequent infection. This susceptibility may be prevented in a number of ways, but also through the use of anti-microbial drugs either as a prophylactic measure for patients such as those undergoing vascular or orthopaedic surgery, or patients who are immunosuppressed. Anti-microbial drugs are more commonly used as a curative measure to combat acquired infection.

The use of anti-microbial drugs should be fully understood to provide effective and appropriate treatment, prior to their use. Selection of the most appropriate drug can be partly achieved through knowledge of the organism responsible for the infection. The classification of bacteria is achieved by their shape (e.g. cocci are spherical, bacilli are rod shaped). Many are also classified by whether they are gram-positive or gram-negative. Gram-positive organisms remain stained with methyl violet after washing with acetone; this reflects differences in the cell walls of the bacteria.

Anti-microbial drugs work in several different ways in order to inhibit bacterial growth. For example:

- nitroimidazoles inhibit nucleic acid synthesis,
- penicillins, cephalosporins and vancomycin inhibit cell wall synthesis,
- aminoglycosides inhibit protein (hence enzyme) synthesis.

Metronidazole (a nitroimidazoles drug) is active against most anaerobic bacteria and some protozoa (i.e. unicellular organisms). It is used in the treatment of post-operative anaerobic infections and peritonitis. Because it has no action against aerobic organisms it is used as a combined treatment with other anti-microbial drugs (see below).

The penicillins are antibiotics made by living microbes rather than by chemical synthesis. Benzylpenicillin is effective against gram-positive organisms, such as staphylococcus aureus, which commonly causes wound infections, pneumonia and septicaemia. In situations where the infection is due to penicillin-resistant staphylococci, flucloxacillin is often used, as it is resistant to penicillinase.

Cefuroxime belongs to the group of cephalosporin antibiotics; it is given by injection and often used as a prophylactic in surgery and in conjunction with metronidazole. It is effective in combating serious infection where other antibiotics are ineffective.

As infections are becoming more resistant to anti-microbial treatments, more powerful drugs are being developed. Vancomycin is a bactericidal antibiotic that is active against most gram-positive organisms. It is important in the treatment of patients with septicaemia or endocarditis caused by methilcillin-resistant staphylococcus aureus (MRSA).

Aminoglycoside drugs such as gentamicin achieve the inhibition of protein synthesis; they are used to treat acute life-threatening gram-negative infections, such as *Pseudomonas aeruginosa*, until antibiotic sensitivity is known (Neal 1997).

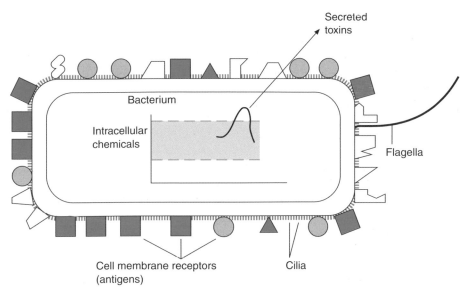

Figure 4.1 The immunogen is the bacterium which may have many
antigens attached to its cell membrane

**Q. Differentiate between the following: an immunogen, an antigen
and a pathogen.**

The aim of this chapter is to highlight the body's natural resistance to trauma, the
body's protective mechanism in response to exposure to pathogens and their
toxins, and to non-microbial antigens, for example incompatible blood cells,
transplanted tissues and organs, and allergic substances (called allergens), for
example chemicals associated with latex.

A more extensive discussion of immunity is provided in other texts (e.g.
Clancy and McVicar 2002). The information provided here and associated reader
texts will enable the reader to complete the activities included in this chapter.

Individuals have different resistances and susceptibilities to infection, depending upon the efficiency of their immunologic response. The subjectivity of an individual's immunological response is governed by a unique genetic ability (inherited
from their biological parents) to respond to harmful agents, and environmental
exposure to potentially harmful agents.

An individual can acquire immunity to infectious disease either naturally or
artificially; both of which can be passive or active. Resistance to infection is comprised of complementary non-specific and specific defence mechanisms (Figure
4.2).

Non-specific immunity is present at birth. These defence mechanisms are the
same for everyone. They are divided into external physico-chemical barriers and
internal (bodily) reactions, including the phagocytic response that provides
immunological surveillance against pathogenic microbes and their toxins.

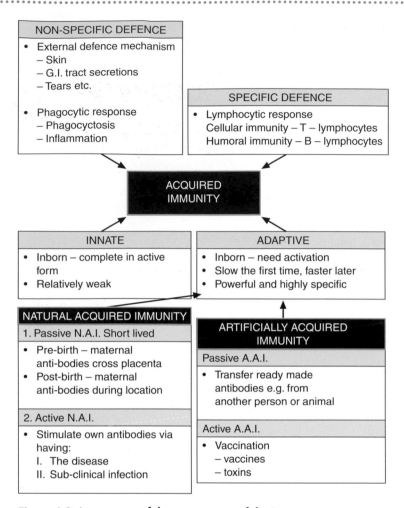

Figure 4.2 **A summary of the components of the immune system**

Q. Which defences, present at birth, provide the body with the defence capability known as the non-specific response?

Specific resistance is the immunity that is acquired during life. It develops mostly after birth when an individual becomes exposed to potential environmental hazards (called antigenic insults). Specific immunity is mediated through a lymphocytic response. It involves the activation of specific lymphocytes (= 'lymph cells') which are stimulated to release their secretions (cytotoxic substances and antibodies) in response to exposure to antigenic substances. Fetuses and neonates receive antibodies from their mothers via the placenta and breast milk, respectively. This passive immunity gives resistance for approximately three months until the transferred antibodies are destroyed. A programme of vaccination is therefore recommended soon after birth, which ensures the acquisition of long-lasting active immunity against pathogens which have the potential to produce serious diseases, such as measles, mumps, diphtheria, whooping cough, tetanus and poliomyelitis.

EXERCISE

Using Figure 4.2 and the relevant sections in your chosen physiology textbook, suggest why some immunization programmes (for example, whooping cough) confer life-long immunity and others (e.g. tetanus) offer relatively short-lived immunity.

Both non-specific and specific immunities are adapted to maintain the equilibrium of the body's internal environment.

The following section is concerned with discussing how external defences are adapted to prevent the entry of antigenic insults into the body, and how internal defences operate once external defences have been breached.

External defence mechanisms

The non-specific components of the external defence mechanisms include skin, mucous membranes, digestive secretions, tears, lysozymes, urination and defecation.

EXERCISE

Before going any further, use Figure 4.3 and a physiology textbook to determine how physico-chemical barriers to infection operate.

Internal defence mechanisms

Non-specific immune responses are also observed inside the body as the inflammatory and phagocytic responses to antigens. Internal defence mechanisms, however, also include the specific immune responses, which act against particular antigens.

Inflammation

Inflammation occurs when cells are damaged. This response has protective and defensive roles, and acts to restore tissue homeostasis by neutralizing and destroying antigens at the site of injury. Inflammation, being non-specific, involves the same response to all antigenic insults and tissue injury.

The degree of inflammation depends upon the extent of tissue damage and the microbe's pathogenicity (i.e. the ability to cause disease).

These factors together with the stages of inflammation and the physiology of wound healing are discussed later in this chapter.

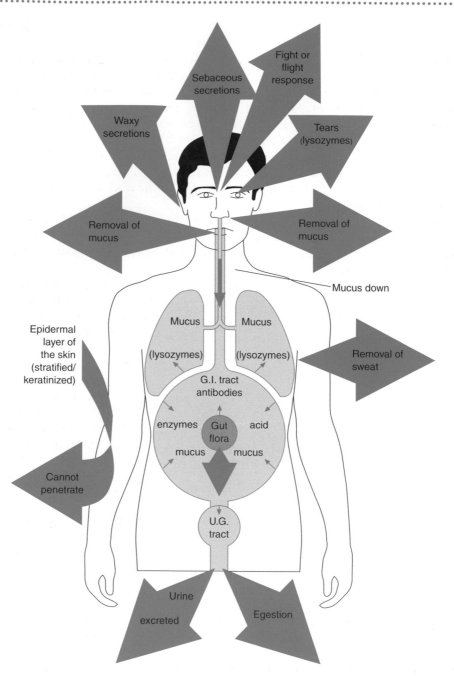

Figure 4.3 **The physical and chemical barriers of natural immunity**
(G.I., Gastrointestinal, U.G., Urinary-genital)

Q. Describe how the pH of the gastrointestinal tract is related to providing immunity.

Phagocytosis

Microbes that have penetrated the external defences must be kept in check by internal defence mechanisms. Phagocytosis is the first line of cellular defence against microbial invasion. The process is sometimes so efficient that microbes are removed as potential sources of infection before the lymphocytes have become aware of their presence. Phagocytes exist as microphages and macrophages (micro- = small; macro- = large).

Microphages (e.g. neutrophils and eosinophils) are white blood cells that circulate and police the body by entering injured peripheral tissues. Neutrophils have the greater phagocytosing capacity, since they are more abundant and more mobile than eosinophils.

Macrophages are classified as 'wandering' or 'fixed' monocytes. The former migrate to areas of infection; the latter, for example, Kupffer cells of the liver, are permanent residents of specific tissues. However, these cells can be transported to nearby damaged tissue.

Before phagocytosis begins, mobile microphages and macrophages must move through capillary walls to the vicinity of antigenic material. As a matter of convenience, the process of phagocytosis is divided into four stages summarized in Figure 4.4. Phagocytosis is enhanced if the antigens are coated with specific antibodies, and further improved by the presence of complement proteins (see Figure 4.5).

Microorganisms are not entirely defenceless against phagocytic cells; for example, some microbial toxins kill phagocytes. Other microbes (e.g. tuberculin bacilli) divide within phagocyte vacuoles and destroy phagocytes intracellularly, whilst others (e.g. HIV) remain dormant within phagocytes before exerting their influence. Problems can arise if phagocytosed antigens cannot be 'digested' (e.g. asbestos), thereby accumulating inside the cell. Phagocytes contain an abundance of intracellular organelles called lysosomes, which fuse with the vacuolated particle in an attempt to destroy them. Eventually, phagocytic autolysis ('self-destruction') occurs when the powerful enzymes (called lysozymes) are released inside cells from the lysosomes.

The specific immune response

The non-specific mechanisms have stereotypical action against all antigens. In addition to surviving the non-specific defences, pathogens must also simultaneously deal with specific (lymphocytic) immune defences if they are to be effective in producing infection or disease.

Lymphocytic responses confer immunity against particular antigens. Such responses have two closely allied components, T- and B-lymphocytes.

■ Specific T-lymphocytes attach themselves to antigens to destroy them. This response is particularly effective against the antigens of fungi, intracellular viruses, parasites, foreign tissue transplants and cancer cells. This is called cell-mediated immunity, since it is mainly reliant upon the secretions of cytotoxic T-cells and other substances that influence other cells of the immune system, including macrophage-attracting substances and interferon.

■ B-lymphocytes produce specific antibodies in an attempt to destroy a particular antigen, i.e. antibody X is produced if antigen X penetrates the external defences, whereas antibody Y is produced if antigen Y enters the body. These cells confer humoral (antibody-mediated) immunity, which is particularly effective against bacteria and viral antigens.

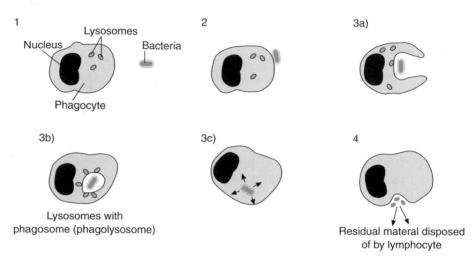

Figure 4.4 **Phagocytosis**
1 Chemotaxis – chemical attraction via microbial toxins
2 Adhesion
3a Ingestion
3b Intracellular digestion
3c Intracellular absorption of useful products
4 Disposal.

Q. Phagocytes move through capillary walls by squeezing between adjacent endothelial. This process is known as:
a adhesion,
b chemotaxis,
c perforation,
d diapedesis.

EXERCISES

1 Using a nursing dictionary make notes on the following:
   cytotoxic, antibody, passive immunity, active immunity, diphtheria, tetanus, poliomyelitis, post-operative infection and meningitis
2 Prior to considering cell-mediated and antibody-mediated reactions, readers should use a physiology textbook to familiarize themselves with the embryological origin of T- and B-cells.

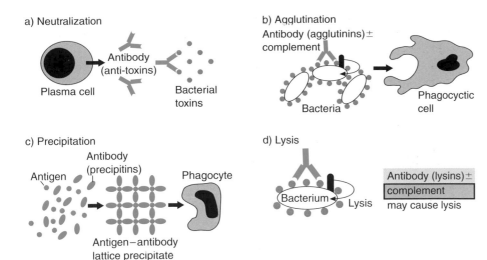

Figure 4.5 **Antibody–antigen complexing**

a   Antibody = anti-toxin,
b   Antibody = agglutinin,
c   Antibody = precipitin,
d   Antibody = lysin.

Q. Complement activation:

a   attracts phagocytes,
b   enhances phagocytosis,
c   stimulates inflammation,
d   all the above.

In adults, mature lymphocyte production occurs in the bone marrow and lymphatic tissue. Lymphocytes have long lifespans compared with most body cells; approximately 80 per cent survive four years, and some live for twenty years or more. Lymphocyte production must match their destruction to maintain the homeostatic functions of the immune system. The ageing process is associated with increased destruction and decreased production rates. It is, therefore, not surprising that the elderly are more susceptible to infection and disease.

Activating the lymphocytic response

Very few antigens appear to bind directly to antigen-reactive T- or B-lymphocytes. Instead some are presented to the lymphocytes on the surface of the macrophages following phagocytosis. These are termed antigen-presenting cells (APCs) (Figure 4.6).

An important group of APCs is the non-phagocytic dendritic cells. These cells are widely distributed, and appear to trap the antigen, thereby preventing its spread. They then initiate local immune responses. Dendritic cells of the lymph nodes and spleen trap circulating antigens in the lymph and blood, presenting them to the resident lymphocytes. Immunogenic human antigens, such as those associated with incompatible blood transfusions, transplanted organs, cancers or 'self' antigens that have changed, also sensitize T-lymphocytes.

Upon contact with an antigen, the macrophages secrete a chemical called inter-leukin-1 (a cytokine) which is responsible for promoting lymphoidal T- and B-cell production. This proliferation stimulates further macrophage activity and hence further proliferation (i.e. a positive feedback mechanism in operation). Macro-phages, dendritic cells, T- and B-lymphocytes thus co-operate with one another to provide immunity against antigenic insults (Figure 4.6).

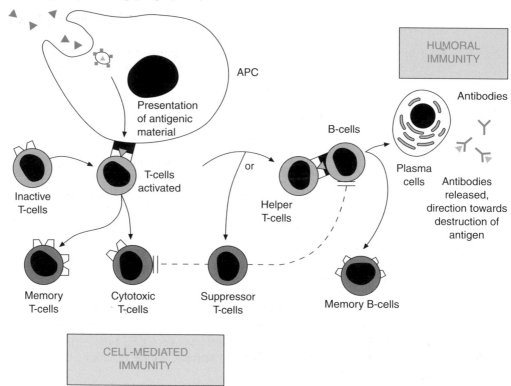

Figure 4.6 Interactions between macrophages, T-cells and B-cells. Non-phagocytic dendritic cells also present antigenic material to activate the lymphatic response. APC – Antigenic-presenting cell

Q. How would a lack of T-helper cells affect the humoral mediated immune response?

> **Box. 4.2   Application: palpation of lymph nodes – a sign of infection!**
>
> A lymph node under antigenic stimulation shows T- and B-cell multiplica-
> tion, and becomes enlarged in the process; the cervical, axillary or inguinal
> lymph nodes are often palpated during medical examination to indicate the
> presence/absence of infection.

Cell-mediated immunity (activating T-lymphocytes)

There are thousands of different T-cells, but only those specifically programmed
to react with the particular antigen present are activated. Sensitized T-lymphocytes divide (Figure 4.6), giving rise to the following *clones* (identical cells).

Killer (cytotoxic) T-cells

The stimulation of killer T-cells is known as cell-mediated immunity, since killer
cells attach themselves to immunogenic antigens and kill foreign cells (immunogens) by secreting the following cytotoxic substances:

i   amplify inflammatory and macrophage responses.

i   cytotoxins. Causing immunogen lysis.
ii cytokines. These provide most of the protection granted by killer cells but act
    in a variety of ways. Cytokines include:
    ■ transfer factors. These recruit lymphocytes by transforming non-sensitized
      T-lymphocytes into sensitized T-cells.
    ■ macrophage-chemotaxic factor. This chemical attracts macrophages, thus
      intensifying phagocytosis.
    ■ macrophage-activating factor. These factors directly increase the phago-
      cytic activity of macrophages.
    ■ migration inhibitory factor. This chemical prevents the migration of
      macrophages, thus encouraging their presence at the site of infection.
iii interferon. This antiviral agent prevents viral replication in infected cells.
    Thus, since antibodies cannot enter cells, interferon succeeds where anti-
    bodies fail! Interferon also enhances killer cell activity, which results in the
    destruction of the host cells.
iv lysozymes. These enzymes (i.e. carbohydrases, proteases, lipases and nucle-
    ases) have the potential to lyse all immunogenic material.

Helper T-cells

Helper lymphocytes assist plasma cells (those derived from B-lymphocytes) to
secrete antibodies. In addition, helper cells secrete interleukin-2, a chemical that

amplifies the multiplication of killer cells. However, interleukin-2 must be activated by interleukin-1, secreted from macrophages, thus demonstrating the interdependency of leucocytes in controlling the homeostatic functions of defence. Interleukins also:

i   amplify inflammatory and macrophage responses,
ii   elevate body temperature, interfering with the rate of bacterial cell multiplication,
iii aid scar tissue formation by increasing fibroblast activity during wound healing,
iv   promote the release of cortisol,
v   stimulate mast cell (basophil) production (i.e. cells which secrete histamine in response to antigens).

Suppressor T-cells

Suppressor lymphocytes restrain killer cell and B-cell activities, and so help to moderate responses. This is important as they limit the effect of cytotoxic secretions on 'self' tissue in the locality.

The interaction between suppressor and helper T-cells, therefore, regulates the immune response. The ratio of these cells can be used to indicate the presence or absence of infection, and the stage of infection. For instance, a 2:1 ratio of helper to suppressor T-cell occurs when there are no signs of infection. Early in the infection cycle, however, a higher ratio of helper cells (hence, killer cells, B-cells and their antibodies) exists which promote the removal of non-self antigens. Conversely, several weeks later, a high suppressor to helper cell ratio (hence killer and plasma B-cells and their antibodies) is observed. This response declines, as the body's defence mechanisms are successful in destroying the antigenic components i.e. the person is recovering from the infection.

Memory T-cells

Memory cells retain the ability to recognize previously encountered non-self antigens, so that second and subsequent exposures lead to a rapid 'secondary' immune response. Immunity of this kind is thus conferred for a long time, often for life. Production of memory cells in response to administered antigens forms the basis of vaccination programmes.

EXERCISE

Identify the functions of killer, suppressor and helper T-cells.

Antibody or humoral mediated immunity (activating – B-lymphocytes)

The body contains thousands of specialized B-cells, which express on their cell membrane antibodies that act as receptor sites for antigens. Each antibody is capable of responding only to a specific antigen. When a B-cell is exposed to an antigen, small B-lymphocytes (influenced by interleukin from activated macrophages) become larger plasma cells. These produce and secrete into the blood and lymph specific antibodies of the same type as that expressed originally on the surface of the parent cell (even though B-cells remain in lymph). The antibodies then circulate to the site of antigenic invasion.

Antibodies, also called immunoglobulins (Igs), are given Greek letters and include IgG (Ig gamma), IgA (Ig alpha), IgM (Ig mu), IgD (Ig delta) and IgE (Ig epsilon). The structure and homeostatic function of immunoglobulins are summarized in Table 4.1. Antibodies are produced and secreted in response to the presence of antigens. They appear in all bodily tissues, although more are found within blood.

EXERCISE

Using a physiology textbook identify (via ticking the appropriate box in Table 4.2) the specific immunoglobulins which are toxins, agglutinins, precipitins and lysins.

Being proteins, most antibodies consist of two pairs of polypeptide chains, comprised of a pair of 'heavy' (H) chains (i.e. greater than 400 amino acids), and a pair of 'light' (L) chains (approximately 200 amino acids – see Table 4.1, IgG). The partner of each pair is identical; thus an antibody consists of identical halves, joined by disulphide (sulphur–sulphur) bonds. Each half consists of a heavy and a light chain, also held together by disulphide bonds. Within each chain there are two distinct regions:

1   a constant region. This is identical in the number, type and sequencing of its amino acids in all antibodies of the same class; however, this region differs between antibody categories, and is thus responsible for distinguishing between the different types of antibodies and their biological functions.
2   a variable region. This differs for each antibody, even those of the same category, allowing antibodies to recognize and specifically attach themselves to particular antigens. The combining site, at which the antibody molecule combines with the antigen, is a small area of the variable region.

The antibody's combining sites react with antigens in a variety of ways to form large antibody–antigen complexes that neutralize, agglutinate, precipitate or lyse the antigen (Figure 4.5). Other combining sites of the antibody prevent the adhesion necessary for microbes to penetrate the skin and mucous membranes. For example, IgAs in mucus, sweat and digestive secretions coat bacteria, decreasing their capacity for attachment to body surfaces, thus minimizing their penetration of our external defences.

Table 4.1 The structure and homeostatic functions of antibodies

Class	Basic structure	Homeostatic function
IgG		**Monomer** Protects extravascular compartments from microorganisms and their toxins
IgM		**Pentamer** Effective first line of defence against microorganisms in the blood stream. If present at birth suggest intra-uterine infection, e.g. syphilis
IgA		**Dimer** Protects mucosal surfaces
IgD		**Monomer** May influence B-lymphocyte functions
IgE		**Monomer attached to basophils** Protects against intestinal parasites, responsible for many of the symptoms of allergy

Table 4.2 Immunoglobulins classification depending upon antibody–antigen complexing (activity)

	IgG	IgM	IgA	IgD	IgE
Antitoxins					
Agglutinins					
Precipitins					
Lysins					

Within the plasma cell's lifespan (for 5 days to a few weeks), they are capable of producing approximately 2000 antibody molecules per second; their high metabolic rate explains their brief existence. Some B-cells do not possess the genetic capability to differentiate immediately. These are memory B-cells, which together with memory T-cells are programmed to recognize an antigen on its second and subsequent invasion of the body. They are therefore responsible for stimulating the secondary immune response.

Primary and secondary immune responses

Plasma cells initiate antibody production in the primary immune response. The speed of this response is determined by the time it takes for antigenic activation of the appropriate B-cell, and for the multiplication and differentiation of B-cells. Consequently there is a gradual, sustained rise in circulating antibody concentration, peaking approximately one to two weeks after the initial exposure (Figure 4.7). Antibody concentration subsequently declines, assuming that the individual is no longer exposed to those antigens. This decline parallels the death of plasma cells. If one recovers from an infection upon first exposure (without using medication), then it is because the primary response has provided sufficient defence to aid recovery. If, however, the primary response has not provided sufficient defence, then illness is prolonged and medication (e.g. antibiotics) must be used to facilitate recovery.

Memory cells have long lifespans; some survive twenty years, and the secondary (anamnestic, or memory) response occurs immediately on second contact with an antigen during this period, resulting in rapid antibody secretion in large quantities. Peak values are higher and occur more quickly compared with those of the primary response (Figure 4.7). The secondary response is usually so swift that signs or symptoms of the illness do not appear, since the microbe is destroyed quickly and efficiently. However, if signs and symptoms appear, they are often milder than upon first exposure to the antigens; their presence usually infers that the antigen has slightly changed, possibly indicating a pathogenic mutation. The immediate antibody upsurge of the response may itself have pathological consequences, particularly if normal cells are also destroyed by the response, since this could trigger a massive widespread inflammatory response.

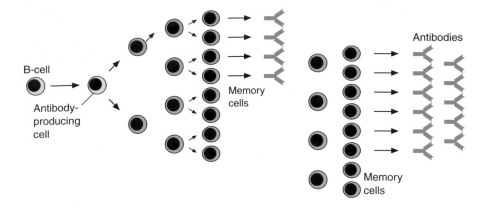

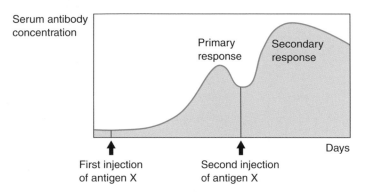

Figure 4.7 **The primary and secondary immune responses**

Q. Identify the principal differences between the primary and secondary immune responses.

The memory or anamnestic response forms the basis of immunization programmes, i.e. the initial immunization sensitizes the body, so that if the immunogen/antigen is encountered in the future through infection, or a booster dose of the antigen is administered, then the body experiences the anamnestic response. Booster dosages are required because antibodies and memory cells have a limited metabolic lifespan and therefore the antigen must be given periodically to maintain high antibody titres.

There is a lag phase between antigen exposure and antibody production. The duration of this phase is largely dependent upon the pathogenicity of the organism concerned; the mode of entry of the organism, and whether the immune response is a primary or secondary response.

Normally, immunogens/antigens stimulate both cellular and humoral immune responses; however, one type usually predominates depending upon the invading immunogen (Figure 4.8).

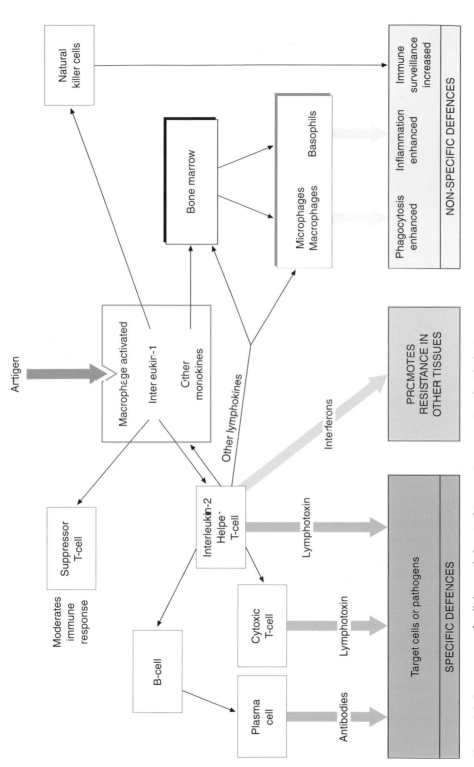

Figure 4.8 A summary of cellular and chemical interactions associated with the immune response

Q. How does the antibody–antigen complex cause elimination of an antigen?

Box 4.3 Application: tissue typing and immunosuppressant therapy

The antigens on erythrocytes are used to categorize one's blood group status. Antigens of other body cells (called histocompatibility antigens) are used to determine an individual's tissue type. Transplanted tissues and organs thus possess non-self antigenic material, and recipients therefore produce cell-mediated and antibody-mediated immune responses against transplanted antigens, which may cause transplant rejection. Tissue typing and immunosuppressant therapy minimize the possibility of rejection.

Tissue typing involves matching the donor and recipient lymphocytic antigens (HLA). Several hundred genes at the HLA loci on chromosome 6 determine histocompatibility antigens. A great variation of HLAs therefore exists since there are thousands of possible genetic, and thus antigenic, combinations; a complete match is extremely unlikely. The closer the HLA match between donor and recipient, the greater the likelihood of transplant success and a nationwide computerized registry assists in this process. Doctors select the most histocompatible and needy organ transplant recipients whenever donor organs become available. Despite national and international co-operation to match donors with recipients, immune rejection is still the main hazard in transplantation. Tissues with a similar genetic make-up are less likely to be rejected. Thus:

1 autograft (graft from the person's own body tissues), having no non-self-antigens, is obviously not rejected.
2 isograft (grafting from individuals with 'identical' genetic make-up, i.e. identical or monozygotic twins) have little risk of rejection.
3 allograft or homograft (grafting between members of the same species, but not genetically identical individuals) has a higher rate of rejection.
4 xenograft or heterograft (using a graft from a different species) has the highest rate of rejection.

Immunosuppressant drugs are also of value in treating people with severe hypersensitivity states, autoimmune conditions and to minimize the risk of transplant rejection. These drugs are aimed at T-lymphocytes, since these cells are the most active in rejection. Unfortunately, immunosuppressants are non-specific, and suppression of the patient's natural defences, to otherwise trivial pathogens, may result in infection or disease, which may threaten the life of the recipient. For example:

■ corticosteroids (e.g. prednisolone and hydrocortisone) are used for preventing transplant rejections, in the treatment of severe allergies and for autoimmune conditions. They operate by gradually destroying lymphoidal tissue, which directly depletes T- and B-cells. Their main action, however, is to decrease the activities of phagocytic cells. Thus, they may make recipients more susceptible to infections.

- cytotoxic drugs (e.g. methotrexate and 6-mercaptopurine) are used to inhibit replication of lymphocyte mitosis. In addition, however, they also inhibit mitosis of other cells, for example in the bone marrow, gastrointestinal tract and skin cells. Consequently, these drugs can produce undesirable side effects, such as thrombocytopenia, anaemia, leucopenia, hair loss, skin disorders, and gastrointestinal upsets.
- the drug cyclosporine inhibits secretion of interleukin-2 by helper T-cells but only has a minimal effect on B-cells. Thus, the risk of rejection is diminished while retaining resistance to some diseases.
- anti-lymphocytic serum (ALS) depletes T-cells, but also damages other lymphocytes, making a recipient more susceptible to infection. Immunizing horses or rabbits with human lymphocytes produces the serum. However, it has a limited use in preventing the rejection of transplanted organs.

EXERCISE

Using information from this chapter reflect on your understanding by differentiating between:

- the specific and non-specific immune responses,
- the specialized and distinctive roles of T- and B-lymphocytes,
- the primary and secondary immune responses.

An overview of the homeostatic responses involved in wound healing

Wound healing is a remarkable process and without it surgery would be impossible. However, even today, relatively little is known regarding the mechanisms involved or the factors that influence it. Furthermore, as surgery advances, wound healing becomes more significant. Patients with systemic ischaemia, infection, pre-existing medical conditions such as jaundice and diabetes mellitus, malnutrition and those taking anti-inflammatory and steroidal drugs – the problems are numerous, but the requirement is the same; that is, a safely healed wound when surgery is complete.

Wound assessment has traditionally been the responsibility of nursing staff and has tended to be subjective, often relying on anecdotal evidence, which frequently fails to report accurate information (Flanagan 1996). Accurate wound assessment and management is dependent on an understanding of the physicobiochemistry of healing and the factors that delay this process, as well as the optimal conditions required at the wound surface to maximize healing.

This chapter illustrates the homeostatic responses to injury and, hopefully, may stimulate interest in this neglected area of study.

A wound may be defined as:

An interruption to the continuity of the external and/or internal surface of the body, which may be due to accidental injury, planned surgery, thermal injury, pressure, or disease process such as leg ulceration or carcinoma.

(Clancy and McVicar 2002)

The extent of tissue injury and/or tissue death (necrosis) is largely dependent on the intensity and duration of the exposure to the injurious agent, as well as the type of tissue involved. Extremes of temperature, for example, denature enzymes, consequently compromising the structural and functional integrity of cellular organelles and thus damaging cells due to glucose utilization becoming severely reduced (Clancy and McVicar 2002).

The homeostatic responses of tissue repair, regeneration and replacement are necessary following tissue injury and/or tissue death to maintain the number of cells within their homeostatic limits, and thus to not compromise cellular, tissue, organ and organ system homeostatic functional integrity. Tissues can be divided into three categories according to their homeostatic responses (see Figure 4.9).

The first chapter discussed the importance of the interdependency of organ systems in maintaining intracellular homeostasis. This interdependence is vital in producing the optimal physicobiochemical conditions required at the wound surface to maximize the healing process. For example:

■ efficient digestive functioning provides essential intracellular nutrients (metabolites and products of metabolism) for repair, regeneration of cells and restoration of tissue structural and functional integrity following injury (see Table 4.3, Figure 4.10 and pp. 119–24 on stages of wound healing).

■ efficient circulatory working is necessary to transport white cells (to protect the integrity of the undamaged cells), nutrients, oxygen and biochemicals important to the wound healing process to the site of tissue damage.

■ the lymphatics prevent the excessive accumulation of tissue fluid via drainage, in order to minimize the discomfort and/or pain that can accompany inflammation as a result of fluid compression within surrounding soft tissues.

■ excretory organs remove self and non-self-cellular/chemical debris from the damaged site which otherwise would increase the incidence of septicaemia and toxaemia, particularly during injury accompanied by an infection.

■ the co-ordinators (neural/hormonal mediators) of body function direct the systemic interactions involved in providing the optimal physicobiochemical conditions for the wound healing process.

It is evident, therefore, that an inefficiency (or homeostatic imbalance) of one component leads to functional disturbance of other parts of the body. For example, if cardiovascular function is compromised (e.g. through progressive atherosclerosis), wound healing is delayed due to an inadequate cardiovascular homeostatic response to tissue damage.

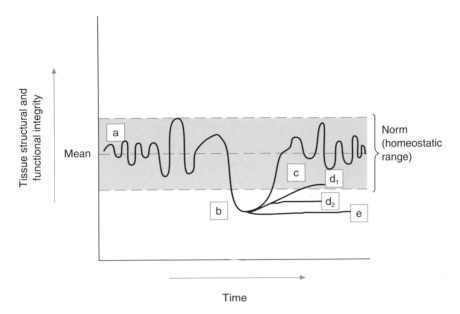

Time

Figure 4.9 **Repair, regeneration and restoration of a tissue's structural and functional integrity following injury**

a Structural and functional integrity of body tissues intact.

b Compromised structural and functional integrity of the body's tissues due to tissue loss.

c A speedy and complete repair and regeneration with complete restoration of the functional integrity of body tissues. Labile tissues, such as the skin, undergo mitosis throughout life and therefore have such excellent repair capabilities.

d_1/d_2 A complete or partial repair and regeneration with only a partial restoration of the functional integrity of body tissues following injury. Stable tissues, such as the liver, normally exhibit little mitotic activity during adult life but are capable of increasing the rate of cell division if they are damaged. Although such tissues may heal, their complex architecture may not regenerate and they may not necessarily be restored to full function.

e Minor repair and regeneration with a loss of functional integrity of tissue following injury, resulting in scarring of the damaged area. Permanent tissues such as the brain, spinal cord and skeletal muscle exhibit little mitotic activity during adult life. They are so complex that little repair other than scarring can be achieved following injury.

Table 4.3 Role of nutrients in the process of wound healing. Note that nutrients are intracellular metabolites and/or products of metabolism

Intracellular metabolites/ products vital for wound healing process		Role of nutrients in providing intracellular products vital for wound healing	Nutrient deficiency: the effect on wound healing
Macronutrients			
Proteins			
General role of proteins		Metabolism of cell membranes Enzymes synthesis	Prolonged inflammation Impairs fibroplasia
Specific roles of some amino acids	Cysteine	Important role in collagen synthesis	Delays collagen synthesis Delays angiogenesis Delays wound remodelling
	Argenine	Enhanced collagen synthesis Enhances immune response	Weaker wounds
Lipids			
General roles of lipids		Concentrated energy source Metabolism of cell membranes	Rare
Specific role of a fatty acid	Linoleic acid	Maintains integrity and function of cellular unit membranes Prostaglandin precursor	Rare
Carbohydrates			
General role of carbohydrates		Energy source for all cells	
Specific role of glucose		Primary energy fuel for metabolism of leucocytes and fibroblasts	Gluconeogenesis from protein metabolism resulting in protein – energy malnutrition in patients with severe injuries

Table 4.3
Continued

Micronutrients

Vitamins

General role of vitamins		Co-factors therefore important for general metabolism and maintenance of health	
Specific roles of some vitamins	Vitamin C	Co-factor for several amino-acids Anti-oxidant factor enhances wound healing	Wounds healing inefficiently Increase likelihood of pressure sore development
	Vitamin B complex	Involved in collagen cross linkages	Rare
	Vitamin A	Epithelial proliferation/migration *Collagen cross linkages	Rare
	Vitamin E	Anti-oxidant may work with Vitamin C	Rare

Minerals

General role of minerals	Co-factors therefore important for general metabolism and maintenance of health	
Specific roles of minerals		
Iron (Fe)	*Co-factor important in collagen synthesis	Anaemia therefore delays the wound healing process Decreased collagen synthesis/cell proliferation
Zinc (Zn)	*Co-factor important in collagen synthesis, protein synthesis	Decreased wound healing processes
Copper (Cu)	*Co-factor important in collagen cross linkages	
Calcium (Ca)	*Remodelling of collagen	
Magnesium (Mg)	*Synthesis of collagen	

Note
*Therefore strengthening scars important in remodelling of collagen, thus deficiencies lead to decreased collagen cross linkages. This reduces the strength of scar tissue.

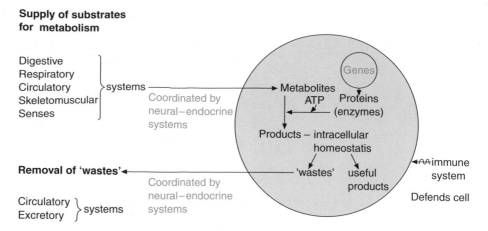

Supply of substrates for metabolism

Figure 4.10 **The interdependency of organ systems in providing intracellular metabolites and products necessary for wound healing**

Intracellular metabolites include: micronutrients (see Table 4.3)
Intracellular products include: macronutrients (see Table 4.3) and products of metabolism which are important in the healing process. These include:

- serotonin (released from basophils),
- histamine (released from basophils),
- platelets and cells that have been damaged,
- prostaglandins and kinins (released from cells that have been damaged),
- clotting factors (released from cells that have been damaged and platelets),
- antibodies (released from B-lymphocytes),
- collagen and elastin (released from fibrocytes),
- macrophage-attracting substances such as compliment (released from liver cells),
- prothrombin and fibrinogen (released from liver cells),
- cytotoxic substances (released from T-lymphocytes),
- mitotic growth factors (released from cells, which have no contact inhibition).

Q. From the list above identify pain-producing chemicals.

EXERCISE

Which of the following is correct?

Septicaemia is a condition where:

a there is formation of secondary abscesses due to the presence of septic foci.
b transient bacteria are present in the blood stream.
c actively multiplying bacteria are present in the blood stream.
d staphylococcus aureus is present in the tissues.

See the end of this chapter for the answer

Local and general responses to injury

The homeostatic responses to injury can be conveniently divided into local responses (those in the injured tissues) and general responses (those elicited in the rest of the body by the local response). The latter can be referred to as 'shock'. Many forms of shock exist, each of which describe the pattern of responses to a particular injury or 'antigenic (non-self) insult': for example, cardiogenic shock (response to heart failure), haemorrhagic shock (response to haemorrhage), traumatic shock (response to trauma) and septic or endotoxic shock (response to infection).

EXERCISE

Review the discussion on types of shock in Chapter 5 and revise the pre-operative and post-operative measures used to prevent shock.

Wound healing does not, of course, only apply to the skin, though the skin is more susceptible to damage than the underlying tissues (see Chapter 2, 'The surgical approach', p.28). Other tissue, for example muscles, may be torn, bones fractured and blood flow disrupted during a major surgical procedure such as open-heart surgery; this chapter considers the healing of skin wounds only.

EXERCISE

Before continuing, the reader is advised to review the structure of the skin in Chapter 2.

Classification of wounds

Wounds are conventionally classified as superficial (or non-bleeding) and deep (or bleeding). Damage to the epidermis will not result in bleeding since this layer does not contain blood vessels; its main function is to form a protective covering from the external environment. Wound healing of this tissue, for example after mild abrasion, involves only the replacement of cells known as the germinal layer, since the layers above it are derived from the cell division within this layer of cells (Figure 4.11a).

Damage to the deeper dermal layer results in a bleeding wound since the blood vessels are present in this cutaneous layer of the skin (Figure 4.11b). This type of injury involves a more complicated type of wound healing. The first set of homeostatic responses involved are repair and regeneration of damaged blood vessels to restore their role of transportation of the vital factors essential for the healing of the damaged tissue, i.e. epidermal cells. Of course, if blood vessels are directly damaged and ruptured, blood will be lost at the site of the injury, either escaping to the outside or being retained in the tissue as a bruise or haematoma.

Wound classification may be clean, bacterially contaminated, or infected.

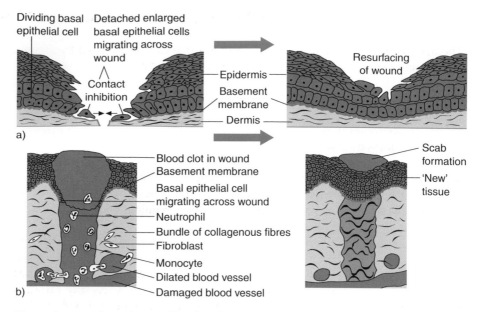

Figure 4.11 **Epidermal wound healing following injury**
a Epidermal wound healing following superficial injury, e.g. a mild abrasion of the skin. Division of basal (germinating) cells and migration across a superficial wound
b Epidermal wound healing following injury to deep layers of the skin, e.g. a surgical incision. Involves generation of a new blood supply (angiogenesis) before the division of and migration of basal (germinating) cells across the surface of the wound.

Box 4.4   Application: healing by primary and secondary intentions

Wound healing of all connective soft tissues occurs in a similar manner, which involves the formation of new epithelium and contraction of healthy granulation tissue beneath (see pp. 129–31), to form a fibrous scar. There are basically two types of wound healing – primary and secondary intentions. Healing by primary intention or closure is the most common type of healing following surgery. It occurs when the tissue edges are maintained in apposition. The lower layers are sutured with a dissolvable suture and the skin is either sutured or clipped together (Plate 4i). This should be achieved in all incised surgical wounds or primarily sutured fresh traumatic lacerations. The wound heals quickly with minimal scarring.

In healing by secondary intention, the wound edges are distant from each other, and the defect fills via granulation tissue from the lowest part of the wound upwards with the epithelial layer being the last to grow (Plate 4ii). This type of wound closure is achieved sometimes in full thickness burns, chronic leg ulceration, after surgical excision of necrotic tissue, following some surgical procedures, for example closure of a fistula-in-ano and pilonidal sinus, and where the wound is infected.

Details of the stages involved in wound healing

The healing process occurs as a set of homeostatic responses initiated by trauma. The process can be conveniently divided into four main stages:

1   the vascular stage,
2   the inflammation stage,
3   the proliferation stage,
4   the maturation stage.

Sub-stages or phases exist within the main stages, for example the platelet and blood coagulation phases of the vascular stage. There is, however, considerable overlap between the stages and phases and the time required by an individual to progress onto the next stage and phase of healing.

Careful assessment by the nurse is vital in identifying the specific stage and phase of the healing process since treatment may vary at each stage and phase (Flanagan 1996). Thus, poor wound management often results from an incorrect identification of the stage of wound healing or a failure to detect any variation from the normal process. Therefore, the characteristics associated with healing are a vital part of the nursing process, and according to Flanagan (1996) nursing clinical observation skills play a fundamental role by identifying the presence of:

- prolonged inflammation,
- infection,
- necrotic tissue,
- unhealthy granulation tissue,
- tissue ischaemia,
- delayed epithelialization,
- skin maceration,
- skin sensitivities and allergies,
- pain,
- poor physical and nutritional status,
- fluid imbalance,
- hypoxia.

EXERCISE

Using a physiology textbook suggest why the composition of blood is important for maintaining intracellular homeostasis, and distinguish between the following terms: whole blood, serum and plasma.

The vascular stage

Seconds after damage to blood vessels, their muscular walls contract. This vascular spasm (called vasoconstriction) decreases blood flow and minimizes blood loss for up to thirty minutes, thus aiding other homeostatic responses within the haemostatic response. Haemostasis is the term used to describe the responses associated with arresting bleeding. In addition to the vascular stage of haemostasis, two further processes act to prevent further blood loss: the platelet and blood coagulation phases (see Figure 4.12).

These mechanisms are adequate as homeostatic controls in preventing blood loss if the damage is to small blood vessels. If larger blood vessels are involved (resulting in massive haemorrhage), however, these mechanisms are inadequate and, as with all homeostatic failures, there will be a need for clinical intervention to correct the imbalance (Clancy and McVicar 2002).

Platelet phase

The platelets (also called thrombocytes) that come into contact with the damaged vessel enlarge, becoming irregular in shape. They become extremely sticky, adhering to the collagen fibres of the vessel wall. These platelets secrete substances, which activate more platelets, causing them to stick to the original ones. The aggregation and attachment of platelets forms a platelet 'plug'; this forms almost immediately after the damage. The plug becomes strengthened by fibrin threads formed during the coagulation process and is, therefore, extremely effective in preventing blood loss from small vessels.

Blood coagulation phase

Coagulation is a complicated metabolic pathway involving many interdependent enzymatically controlled reactions. Collectively these reactions are called the 'clotting cascade' which is a multiplicative process: proenzymes (inactive enzymes) interact, and the conversion of one proenzyme creates an enzyme that activates a second proenzyme that activates a third proenzyme, and so on, in a chain reaction or domino effect. There are many clotting factors involved (see Table 4.4). These include plasma factors (numbered I to XIII), and platelet

---

Figure 4.12 (opposite) **The clotting mechanism**
Details of plasma and platelet clotting factors are discussed in the text, pp. 120–4, and in Table 4.3
1   Vascular phase. Damaged blood vessels go into spasm via contraction of their smooth muscle. This decreases blood flow and thus minimizes blood loss.
2   Platelet phase. Platelets aggregate, accumulate and adhere to the damaged vessels forming a platelet plug.
3   Coagulation phase. Activation of clotting and clot formation.
4   Clot retraction phase. Involves the contraction of the blood clot.
5   Clot destruction phase. Enzymatic (plasmin) destruction of the clot.

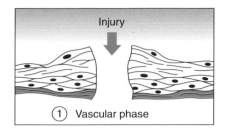

① Vascular phase

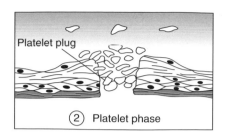

② Platelet phase

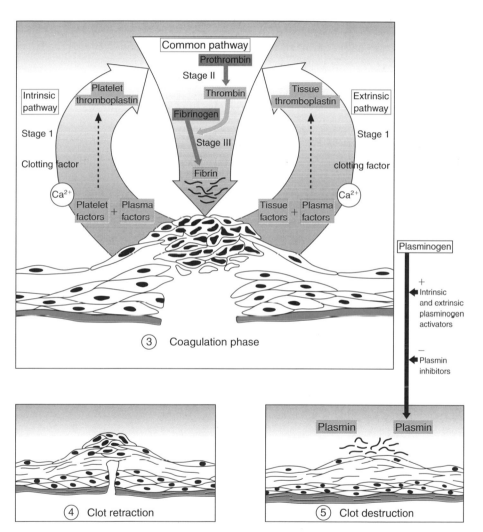

③ Coagulation phase

④ Clot retraction

⑤ Clot destruction

Q. How could an enzyme, such as streptokinase, assist in preventing unwanted clotting and removing clots already formed (see Box 4.5)?

Table 4.4 The homeostatic importance of coagulation factors

Coagulation factors	Homeostatic importance
Plasma coagulation factors	
I Fibrinogen	Important factor in stage III of clotting, in which it is converted to fibrin
II Prothrombin	Important in stage II of clotting in which it is converted into thrombin
III Thromboplastin (or thrombokinase, Prothrombinase)	In extrinsic pathway it is referred to as extrinsic thromboplastin; it is formed from tissue thromboplastin. In the intrinsic pathway it is referred as intrinsic thromboplastin; it is formed from platelet disintegration. Formation of thromboplastin signifies the end of stage I.
IV Calcium ions	Involved in all three stages of clotting. Removal of calcium or its binding in the plasma prevents coagulation
V Proaccelerin (or labile) factor	Required for stages I and II of both extrinsic and intrinsic pathways
VI No longer used in coagulation theory	
VII Serum prothrombin accelerator (or stable) factor	Required in stage I extrinsic pathway
VIII Anti-haemophilic factor	Required for stage I of intrinsic pathway. Deficiency causes haemophilia A
IX Christmas factor (or plasma thromboplastin component)	Required for stage I of intrinsic pathway. Deficiency causes haemophilia B
X Stuart factor (or Stuart-Prower) factor	Required for stages I and II of extrinsic and intrinsic pathways. Deficiency results in nose bleeds, bleeding into joints, or bleeding into soft tissues
XI Plasma thromboplastin antecedent	Required for stage I of intrinsic pathway. Deficiency causes haemophilia C
XII Hageman factor	Required for stages I of intrinsic pathway
XIII Fibrin stabilizing factor	Required for stage III of clotting
Platelet coagulation factors	
Platelet factor 1 (Pf1)	Essentially the same as plasma coagulation factor V
Platelet factor 2 (Pf2)	Accelerates formation of thrombin in stage I intrinsic pathway and the conversion of fibrinogen to fibrin
Platelet factor 3 (Pf3)	Required for stage I of intrinsic pathway
Platelet factor 4 (Pf4)	Binds heparin, an anticoagulant during clotting

Q. What is the outcome of the first, second and third stages of clotting?

Q. Name the vitamin that is required for the synthesis of Factors II (prothrombin), VII, IX and X.

factors (labelled Pf1 to Pf4). This cascade occurs rapidly once stimulated, and when blood is taken, or a vessel damaged, blood is quickly converted from its usual liquefied state into a gel-like clot. The process is initiated within thirty seconds of damage and completed after several minutes. The coagulation phase can be summarized as being a sequence of three stages.

Stage I

The formation and the release of a collection of enzymes collectively called 'thromboplastin' (also called thrombokinase or prothrombinase).

Stage II

Conversion of plasma prothrombin into thrombin via the actions of thromboplastin.

Stage III

Conversion of the soluble protein fibrinogen into insoluble fibrin by the actions of thrombin; the fibrin then forms the threads of the clot.

The 'initiating' enzyme (thromboplastin) is released from damaged cells, triggering the extrinsic coagulation pathway and/or by the lysis of platelets, which triggers the intrinsic coagulation pathway.

Extrinsic pathway

This pathway is initiated by the release of the initiating enzyme from damaged peripheral cells and/or damaged capillary endothelial cells. This enzyme together with certain plasma factors (IV, V, VII and X) forms extrinsic or tissue thromboplastin, which is equivalent to stage I of the clotting cascade. The second stage utilizes extrinsic thromboplastin to convert prothrombin into thrombin. The third stage is promoted with the conversion of fibrinogen into fibrin by the action of thrombin and plasma factors IV and XIII. Most steps in the extrinsic mechanism also require the presence of calcium ions.

Intrinsic pathway

This pathway is activated by a rough surface such as 'fatty' plaques or calcium deposits attached to the internal lining of the blood vessel. This stimulus removes the normal repulsion activities between platelets and endothelial cells lining the blood vessels, with the result that platelets adhere to the rough surface. The aggregation and clumping of platelets bring about their breakdown (called lysis), releasing platelet coagulation factors (Pf1–4) into the plasma. The clumping reaction is sometimes all that is necessary to plug lightly damaged areas.

Stage I of the intrinsic pathway involves four platelet factors (Pf1–4) and seven plasma factors (IV, V, VIII, IX, X, XI, XII) to form intrinsic thromboplastin. The second stage involves the conversion of prothrombin into thrombin by the thromboplastin. The third stage is the same for both intrinsic and extrinsic pathways. All stages of the intrinsic pathway require the presence of calcium ions.

Vitamin K is required for the synthesis of four clotting factors: factors II (prothrombin), VII, IX and X and thus vitamin K deficiency often leads to uncontrolled bleeding.

Thrombin is a key chemical because of its involvement in the third stage and because it stimulates more platelets to adhere to one another, resulting in a further lysis of platelets and thus the consequential release of further platelet factors. The more thrombin that is released, therefore, the more platelet factors are released, resulting in a larger clot formation. This cyclical process is therefore a positive feedback mechanism, which ensures continual platelet lysis until the clot is formed; thus, the healing process can proceed as appropriate.

EXERCISE

Differentiate between negative and positive feedback mechanisms.

Bleeding wounds activate both extrinsic and intrinsic pathways, to maximize clot formation and arrest bleeding. Once thrombin is formed from damaged cells (i.e. the extrinsic pathway) it enhances further production of thrombin (i.e. a positive feedback mechanism) via the intrinsic pathway; whereas damage to the internal lining of blood vessels, for example, caused by an atheromatous plague or calcium accumulation activates the intrinsic pathway.

Once the fibrin meshwork has been formed, the platelets and erythrocytes stick to its strands. The platelets contract with the result that the entire clot retracts, bringing the torn edges closer together and also stabilizing and consolidating the injury. Microfilaments can be observed in the cytoplasm of platelets that is composed of a contractile protein called platelet actomyosin (or thrombosthenin). The clot plugs the damaged vessel to prevent further blood loss and the retraction makes it easier for fibroblasts, smooth muscle cells and endothelial cells to carry out their homeostatic repair functions.

Once the area beneath the clot is repaired, the clot is dissolved via the process of fibrinolysis. This involves activating the plasminogen into the clot, dissolving enzyme plasmin. The process is summarized in Figure 4.12.

EXERCISE

Reflect on your understanding that blood coagulation is an illustration of a positive feedback mechanism working to benefit homeostasis.

Box 4.5 Application: anticoagulant administration in the perioperative period

During the perioperative period drugs are often administered to the patient which are essential to the surgical and clinical treatment of the patient, but may also affect the blood coagulation process. This can cause haemorrhage and lead to delayed wound healing. Infection can also prevent the wound healing process and antibiotic therapy may need to be considered.

The purpose of anticoagulant drugs is to prevent and treat venous thrombosis and embolism. The perioperative phase is often a critical time for the formation of venous thrombosis and embolism. Restricted movements for long periods of time associated with the body's homeostatic response to tissue trauma causing a systemic response (see Chapter 7), and the general physical condition of the patient, increase the risk of developing a thrombosis and ultimately an embolism (see Question, Figure 4.12).

EXERCISE

What is the association between the homeostatic response to tissue trauma and the increased risk of venous thrombosis and embolism?

- Heparin is a short-acting (four to six hours) anticoagulant, which is given intravenously or subcutaneously. The presence of anti-thrombin III (a protease inhibitor in blood) is required in order for heparin to produce its anticoagulant effect; almost immediately it inactivates the thrombin. It is frequently given to patients undergoing vascular surgery, where clot formation within the walls of the arteries at the arterial incision site or the site of anastomosis is common.
- Aspirin is thought to inhibit platelet aggregation and arterial thrombosis. Although it is not given to the patient during the perioperative period, patients who are at risk from myocardial infarction with unstable angina or patients who suffer from thromboembolic disease may be taking aspirin pre-operatively. This can cause an increase in intraoperative bleeding and subsequent delay in the wound healing process. Post-operative anticoagulant therapy can further delay wound healing.
- Warfarin is given orally. It has a delayed effect of two to three days, and therefore heparin is given until the warfarin has attained a therapeutic range. Warfarin is a vitamin K antagonist and lowers the prothrombin concentration in the plasma by inhibiting its synthesis in the liver.

Fibrinolytic drugs are mainly used to dissolve thrombi, which block the coronary arteries in myocardial infarction. Given intravenously they degrade fibrin clots and dissolve thrombi.

The therapeutic effect of these drugs is more effective if given within three hours of myocardial infarction, and is also enhanced when used in conjunction with aspirin. Streptokinase is one of the most commonly used fibrinolytic drugs. It acts by binding to circulating plasminogen forming an activator which then converts any available plasminogen into plasmin which dissolves the clot.

EXERCISES

Which one of the following is correct?

1 Deep vein thrombosis of the calf can be treated by:
   a vitamin K.
   b antibiotic therapy.
   c low protein diet.
   d anticoagulant therapy.

2 A post-operative patient with a diagnosed deep venous thrombosis suddenly develops dyspnoea, chest pain and shock. He is conscious and frightened. Indicate your first priority of action from the following list:
   a administer prescribed heparin and morphine.
   b administer oxygen.
   c reassure patient and place in a comfortable upright position.
   d administer a prescribed oral anticoagulant.

See the end of this chapter for the answers

The inflammation stage

This is part of the non-specific response to infection, noted earlier.

The body reacts in the same way whether a tissue is damaged via mechanical, thermal or chemical causes, or in response to a pathogenic invasion or a hypersensitivity reaction – a latex allergy, for example.

Box 4.6   Application: latex allergy – the people at risk in the perioperative environment

Latex is the sap from the Brazilian rubber tree, hence it is referred to as natural rubber latex (NRL). It contains proteins and resins, and the former cause allergic reactions in sensitive people. Thus the practitioner and patient is at risk in the perioperative environment. Approximately 4 per cent of the UK workforce suffer occupational exposure to NRL, of this group 6 per cent might be at risk of developing a latex sensitivity (Moore 2000).

In the hospital environment powdered gloves are not worn routinely now and they are certainly not used in the sterile environment. The powder acts as a carrier for the latex proteins, hence when powdered gloves are worn more latex protein comes into contact with the skin, where it is subsequently absorbed. Upon removal of the gloves, the powder and proteins are released into the surrounding air where they can be inhaled causing rhinitis, asthma and conjunctivitis. Inhalation and subsequent absorption into the circulation via the mucous membranes present a greater risk of systemic reaction (Charous 2000).

Specific screening for NRL sensitivity should be considered for all patients, although this may be impractical and unrealistic. Therefore consideration must be given for facilitating best practice in the clinical setting. During pre-assessment surgical patients who are high risk of having NRL sensitivity should be offered clinical testing for NRL allergy. All sensitivities and details of their NRL allergy should be documented and all personnel involved in the care of the patient must be informed. Arrangements can then be made for the operating theatre to be cleaned and left free until the patient arrives, and the patient should be the first on the operating list. All equipment used should, as far as possible, be NRL free, although with over 40,000 products in use in the perioperative environment this may not be achievable. Products that are not NRL free must be covered with a barrier material and there should be limited access of staff to the operating theatre. Emergency drugs should also be readily available for use should the patient have an anaphylactic reaction.

In some circumstances such as with emergency patients, the perioperative practitioner may not always have prior knowledge that the patient is NRL sensitive, and these patients could have an anaphylactic reaction to NRL in the perioperative environment; therefore, all equipment used for resuscitation purposes should be latex free. The problem of NRL allergy is growing and manufacturers of medical equipment are now producing latex-free products; however, until there is a totally NRL-free perioperative environment, the perioperative practitioner must minimize the risk of sensitization for patients and colleagues by following their local policy and guidelines.

EXERCISES

1 Identify products that are used in your department that contain latex.
2 Identify latex-free products in your department.
3 Identify the latex allergy policy used within your hospital.
4 Prepare a checklist on how to prepare the perioperative environment for a patient with a known latex allergy.

Inflamed tissue soon exhibits the four classic signs (see Plate 4iii) which provide a reassurance that normal homeostatic responses have been activated following injury (DeCruz 1998). These signs are redness, an increase in tissue temperature, swelling and discomfort and/or pain. These signs may be associated with loss of function. The first three responses are attributed to changes in the microcirculation in the injured tissue. The redness (or erythema) is due to vasodilation of arterioles: heat to increased blood flow, and swelling (or oedema) to an increase in the extravascular fluid content of the injured tissues. Post-traumatic oedema is promoted by an increase in microvascular permeability and is therefore formed by exudate.

Permeability changes are a response to the secretion of cellular products of metabolism from the site of injury. For example:

1 histamine – released from mast cells (or basophils), a type of white cell, platelets and damaged cells at the site of injury.
2 serotonin and heparin – released from mast cells.
3 kinins and prostaglandins – released from injured cells.

EXERCISE

Using a physiology textbook, review the functions of the white cell types found circulating in blood and those 'policing' the tissues of the body.

The role of the exudate is to promote the movement of proteins and various phagocytic white cells from the plasma into the wound. Generally, the proteins in the tissue fluid create a colloidal osmotic pressure promoting fluid leakage from plasma, resulting in an accumulation of tissue fluid (Chapter 3). The increased blood flow to the area and the accumulation of fluid in the soft tissues eventually exerts pressure on sensory nerve endings, making the wound feel uncomfortable and/or painful (Flanagan 1996). Specifically, proteins such as prothrombin and fibrinogen stimulate the clotting process – a homeostatic response designed to create a physical protective barrier between the external and internal environments of the body.

The next process of inflammation involves the removal of debris and microorganisms (DeCruz 1998). Phagocytes such as neutrophils and macrophages dispose of damaged tissue cells, foreign material and microorganisms via the process of phagocytosis. This process is facilitated by the presence in the exudate of other white cells, T- and B-lymphocytes and various proteinaceous components collectively called complement, which facilitate the phagocytic and lymphocytic responses as homeostatic processes designed to either prevent or fight infection, if present.

EXERCISE

Review the details associated with the non-specific phagocytic response and the specific lymphocytic responses discussed earlier in this chapter.

To summarize, neutrophils are attracted into an area of tissue damage, usually within a few hours of injury; they are soon followed by macrophages. The activities of lymphocytes essentially cleanse the wound bed. Macrophages secrete growth factors, prostaglandins and complement factors, and, since these chemicals promote healing, these cells are usually present during all stages of wound healing. In clean wounds the inflammatory phase lasts approximately thirty-six hours; in necrotic or infected wounds, the process is prolonged (Flanagan 1996).

The biochemical constitution of the exudate reflects the intensity and duration of the injurious agent. For example:

■ serous exudate has a low protein content. Such exudate indicates that there is superficial and minimal damage, e.g. with blistering of the skin.

■ fibrinous exudate indicates damage of a more intense nature, since this type of wound requires the development of a protective fibrin clot. Such material must be removed to prevent scarring.

■ haemorrhagic exudate has the same biochemical constitution as a fibrinous exudate with the additional presence of red blood cells indicating that blood vessels have been damaged during injury.

■ purulent exudate contains pus (i.e. a mixture of living and dead cells of the body, dead microbes, cell debris such as proteinaceous fibres and bacteria toxins). Accumulation of this exudate is detrimental to the healing process.

Although the process of inflammation is considered beneficial, since it involves homeostatic responses which restore tissue homeostatic integrity by neutralizing and destroying antigens locally at the site of injury, the patient may feel generally unwell. Signs and symptoms may include fever, loss of appetite and tiredness. The process of wound healing may also instigate harmful effects such as:

1   oedema in vital organs, such as the lungs, heart and brain. Cerebral oedema is a common cause of raised intracranial pressures in head injury patients.
2   autolysis (self-destruction) of local body tissues due to the release of lysozymes from the large numbers of phagocytes present in the exudate.
3   complications caused by antigen–antibody complexes lodging in blood vessels.

EXERCISE

Review the different types of antigen–antibody complexing that exists. Refer to Figure 4.5 if you are experiencing difficulty.

The proliferation stage

Following the vascular and inflammatory stages, replacement, repair and regeneration of injured cells need to occur. This stage is referred to as proliferation, during which a wound is filled with new connective tissue. The three processes involved are granulation, contraction and epithelialization.

Granulation

The filling of the wound with tissue during proliferation is usually referred to as granulation and this is illustrated in Figure 4.11b. Initially, this process involves the creation of new capillaries (a process called angiogenesis) in the wound bed so as to support the mitotic activity that provides replacement cells. Angiogenesis is stimulated by the tissue hypoxia created from the disruption of blood flow at the time of injury and possibly by chemicals produced by macrophages. Capillary 'buds' develop from the periphery of the wound and grow into the site at about 0.5 mm/day (Collier 1996). Macrophage activity (derived from the process of inflammation) stimulate the production and multiplication of fibroblasts; these cells migrate along the fibrin threads (produced in the vascular phase), depositing a ground substance initiating the production and secretion of collagen. This substance will ultimately form the scar of the wound.

Box 4.7   Application: circulatory malfunctioning decreases wound healing

The importance of an adequate blood supply in granulation is illustrated by the slow rate of healing induced by circulatory deficiencies in conditions such as diabetes mellitus. Granulation is also slowed in the elderly, partly because of reduced cardiovascular efficiency, but also because rates of cell division and cell metabolism decline with age.

The characteristics of healthy and unhealthy granulation tissue are summarized in Plates 4iv and 4v.

Wound contraction

Following the deposition of connective tissue, some fibroblasts are transformed into fibromyoblasts, possibly under the influence of macrophage factors. These cells congregate at the wound margins and use their contractile properties to pull the edges of the wound together, thus reducing the size of the wound (see Figure 4.12 – clot retraction phase).

EXERCISE

The reader should be able to suggest why wound contraction is not necessary in wounds healing by primary intention.

Wound epithelialization

The proliferation and migration of new epithelial cells occur from the wound edge (in skin, remnants of hair follicles, sweat and sebaceous glands), and across the surface of the wound until the wound is closed during the final stages of healing. Why cells should begin to migrate is not completely understood. It is thought that the loss of contact between neighbouring cells causes the movement, i.e. cell–cell communication is removed (see Figure 4.11a). Movement stops when other cells once more surround the cell, although these cells must be of the same 'type' (cancer cells, for example, appear to lose contact inhibition). Once the migrated cells have formed a new germinating layer, they will divide and new epidermal strata will be formed. Newly formed epithelial cells have a translucent appearance and are usually whitish-pink (Flanagan 1996, see Plate 4vi) and to some degree 'raised' in relation to the surrounding tissue (Collier 1996). The signs of inflammation should subside; therefore, the amount of wound exudate should decrease and become more manageable.

Complete healing is only possible once the epithelial cells have completely bridged the surface of the wound. Any scab over the wound will slough away, and the new epidermis will become toughened by the production of the protein keratin. The whole process will normally occur within twenty-four to forty-eight hours after injury, although epithelialization may continue for up to a year or longer in injuries sustaining substantial tissue loss where healing is via secondary intention. Factors which create the optimal environment for the healing process are discussed in detail elsewhere (pp. 120–4) and some are summarized in Tables 4.3–4.5.

Table 4.5 Optimal environmental conditions at the wound interface to maximize the healing process

Environmental condition at the wound interface	Importance to wound healing
Moisture	Increased epidermal resurfacing
Oxygen	Hypoxia produces lactoacidosis which stimulates angiogenesis
Perfusion rate	Good perfusion is essential to transport nutrients so as to maximize the viability of damaged tissue
Temperature (37°C)	Reduced temperature at the wound interface decreases phagocytosis and mitotic activity of regenerating tissues
pH	Decreased (or acidic) pH prevents infection
Nutrients	See Table 4.3

Q. Why does whole blood fail to clot when calcium ions are removed?

The maturation stage

Once granulation, wound contraction and epithelialization phases are completed the final stage of wound healing – maturation – occurs. In this phase:

- fibrocytes (fibroblasts and fibromyoblasts) begin to disappear,
- collagen fibres become more organized to form a mesh and start to appear similar to the surrounding area in both colour and texture,
- fibrin, or the original clot is removed by the action of plasmin (see Figure 4.12) (DeCruz 1998).

Once the scar tissue matures, its vascularity decreases and the tissue contracts causing the scar to become flatter, paler and smoother. Mature scar tissues are hairless and contain no sebaceous or sweat glands.

Table 4.6 Role of wound dressings in the wound healing process

Type of wound	Dressing	Activity
Exuding	Alginate foam	• Gelling characteristics, which lift off or soak up exudate • Requires a secondary covering dressing
Dry, sloughy	Hydrogel	• Takes up shape of wound • Donates liquid to wound and facilitates autolytic debridement • Can absorb some liquid • Requires secondary dressing
Dry, sloughy, necrotic granulating	Hydrocolloid	• Impermeable dressing facilitating rehydration and autolytic debridement • Promotes granulation
Burns, skin donor sites, leg ulcers, sinus packing	Paraffin impregnated gauze Silicone	• Prevents dressing fibres from adhering to wound

Q. Indentify the wound dressings you are currently using and consider in what way they enhance the wound healing process. Could a more appropriate dressing be considered?

Box 4.8   Application: surgical wound dressings

The choice of surgical wound dressing can be a complicated process; there are many choices of surgical dressings available (Table 4.6). The choice is dependent on many factors; these include:

- the stage of the wound healing process,
- the type of wound,
- the presence of infection.

Guidelines and protocols, which combine scientific evidence and expert opinion, provide the evidence for optimum wound care treatment and quality care. However as Table 4.5 indicates, intracellular metabolites/products are vital for the wound healing process. Below are some examples of surgical wound dressings, which have different properties aiming to enhance the homeostatic activity of the body.

Many surgical wounds will only require a permeable or semi-permeable adhesive dressing. This type of dressing usually has a protective pad which may be impregnated with an antiseptic such as chlorhexadine hydrochloride, with an outer layer that is adhesive to the skin.

Some of the semi-permeable dressings such as Bioclusive™ and Tagerderm™ allow the passage of water vapour and oxygen to the wound but prevent microbes from accumulating at the wound site to provide a moist healing environment. Wounds that are more complex in nature, such as burns, deep open wounds and infected wounds, will require specific wound dressings to provide the optimum environment to facilitate the wound healing process.

Summary

- Immunity is a response to the invasion of the body by non-self-antigens.
- Immunity is characterized by being: xenophobic – it distinguishes self from non-self components; adaptive – it produces a response to an antigenic invasion; highly specific – its response is personal for different antigenic insults; and anamnestic – its memory component allows the occurrence of primary and secondary responses.
- Individuals have different resistances and susceptibilities to infections, depending upon the efficiency of their immunological responses. Attention must not only be given to the level of hygiene/cleanliness of the perioperative area but also the recovery and ward environments.
- Wound healing following injury is a dynamic process involving the precise co-ordination of a number of homeostatic responses at a cellular and biomolecular level. These responses are divided into a number of stages/phases of wound healing.
- Perioperative practitioners need a sound knowledge of the normal physico-biochemistry associated with the healing process in order to maximize the effectiveness of wound care perioperatively.
- There are many factors exerting an influence upon wound healing, and the actions of the perioperative team contribute to this process. Strict adherence to aseptic techniques is just one example.
- The appropriateness of wound dressings depends upon the stage of healing, type of wound and the presence or absence of infection.
- Finally, it is clear from current evidence on latex allergy (Royal College of Nursing Society of Occupational Health Nursing 2000) that initiatives have to be taken to safeguard not only the people who work in the department, but also the people passing through (patients, relatives and other visitors).

Bibliography

British National Formulary (2002) British Medical Association and Royal Pharmaceutical Society of Great Britain. London.

Brown, K. (1999) Care of the latex sensitive patient in theatre. *British Journal of Perioperative Nursing* 9(4): 170–3

Bryant, R. (2000) *Acute and Chronic Wounds Nursing Management, Second Edition.* London: Mosby.

Focusing on a multi-disciplinary approach, this book provides a comprehensive resource for healthcare providers challenged with the care of acute surgical wounds and all types of chronic wounds. This text conveys a comprehensive and up-to-date understanding of the biology, pathophysiology and management of dermal wounds.

Carroll, P. and Celia, F. (2000) What you need to know about latex allergy. *MLO: Medical Laboratory Observer* 32(7): 64–6.

Charous, B.L. (2000) *Update on Occupational Latex Allergy*, American Academy of Allergy, Asthma and Immunology 56th AGM.

Clancy, J. and McVicar, A.J. (eds) (1998) *Nursing Care: A Homeostatic Casebook.* London: Arnold.

Clancy, J. and McVicar, A.J. (2002) *Physiology and Anatomy. A Homeostatic Approach, Second Edition.* London: Arnold.

Clancy, J., McVicar, A.J. and Cox, J. (2001) Lextex allergy. *British Journal of Perioperative Nursing* 11(5): 222–7.

Clancy, J., McVicar, A.J. and Muncaster, D. (2001) Wound healing and wound healing assessment. *British Journal of Perioperative Nursing* 11(8): 362–700.

Collier, M. (1996) The principles of optimum wound management. *Nursing Standard* 10(43): 22–6.

Davis, B.R. (2000) Perioperative care of patients with latex allergy. *AORN Journal* 72(1): 47–56, 58–62.

DeCruz, G. (1998) The case of a man with a surgical wound. Case study cited in Clancy and McVicar (1998).

Duquesnoy, R.J. (1999) Immunopathology. Histocompatibility testing in organ transplantation. *Laboratory Medicine* 30(12): 796–802.

Dyke, M. (1999). Latex sensitivity and allergy: fact and fiction. *British Journal of Perioperative Nursing* 9(4): 165–8.

Fell, C. (2000). Health and safety series: hand washing. *British Journal of Perioperative Nursing* 10(9): 461–5.

Fenwick, M.J. and Muwanga, C.L. (2000) Anaphylaxis and monoamine oxidase inhibitors – the use of adrenaline. *Journal of Accident & Emergency Medicine* 17(2): 143–4.

This paper examines a case study that highlights the uncertainty regarding the use of adrenaline (epinephrine) in the context of concurrent MAOI use.

Flanagan, M. (1996) A practical framework for wound healing assessment 1: physiology. *British Journal of Nursing* 5(22): 1391–7.

Ford, D.A. and Koehler, S.H. (2001) A creative process for reinforcing aseptic techniques in practices. *AORN Journal* 73(2): 446–50.

This article describes the process used to address perioperative practice issues in aseptic technique.

Haynes, L.C. and Ludgar, J. (2001) Clinical issues. Latex allergy: implications for nurse educators. *Nurse Educator* 26(2): 57–8.

Kaye, E.T. (2000) Topical wound care management. Acute surgical wound care 1: an overview of topical antibacterial agents. *Infectious Disease Clinics of North America* 14(2): 321–39.

Kent, S. (2000) Research focus: antiseptic skin preparation revisited. *British Journal of Perioperative Nursing* 10(7): 364–72.

McConnell, E.A. (1999) Clinical do's and don'ts. Proper hand washing technique. *Nursing* 29(4): 26.

Hand washing is the cornerstone of infection control. McConnell in this article states that following the technique expressed in this paper it is necessary to minimize the spread of pathogens.

May, D. (2000) Infection control. *Nursing Standard* 14(28): 51–9.

Moore, A. (2000) *Latex Allergy.* Oxford: Bandolier Internet Publications.

Moore P. and Foster L. (1998a) Acute surgical wound care 1: an overview of treatment. *British Journal of Nursing* 7(18): 1101–2, 1104–6,

Moore, P. and Foster, L. (1998b). Acute surgical wound care 2: the wound healing process. *British Journal of Nursing* 7(19): 1183–4, 1186–7.

National Association of Theatre Nurses (1997) *Universal Precautions and Infection Control in the Perioperative Setting.* Harrogate: NATN.

Reflecting current theory and research based practice related to universal precautions and infection control, this document provides background information on the emergence of blood-borne pathogens as a risk to healthcare workers.

National Association of Theatre Nurses (1998) *Principles of Safe Practice in the Perioperative Environment.* Harrogate: NATN.

National Association of Theatre Nurses (2000) *Back to Basics.* Harrogate: NATN.

This book covers the core issues that affect every perioperative practitioner on a daily basis. The topic of hand washing is of particular relevance to this chapter.

National Association of Theatre Nurses (2000) *Understanding Latex in the Perioperative Setting.* Harrogate: NATN.

This book is a detailed document that has everything you need to know about latex in the perioperative setting.

Neal, M.J. (1997) *Medical Pharmacology at a Glance, Third Edition.* Oxford: Blackwell Science.

Norfolk Health (1996) *Wound Care Guidelines.* Unpublished work.

Pace, B. (2000) JAMA patient page. Suppressing the immune system for organ transplants. *JAMA: Journal of the American Medical Association* 283(18): 24–84.

Palmer, J. (2000) Organ transplants. *Physiotherapy Frontline* 6(1): 16.

Patel, S.R., Urech, D. and Werner, H.P. (1998) Surgical gowns and drapes into the 21st century. *British Journal of Perioperative Nursing* 8(8): 27–37.

Pearson, T. (2000) The wearing of facial protection in high risk environments. *British Journal of Perioperative Nursing* 10(3): 163–6.

Pinney, E. (2000) Back to basics: hand washing. *British Journal of Perioperative Nursing* 10(6): 328–31.

Rhodes, A. (2000) Latex allergy awareness and protocol. *British Journal of Perioperative Nursing* 10(3): 157–62.

Royal College of Nursing Society of Occupational Health Nursing (1996) *The Avoidance and Management of Latex Glove Allergy: A Practical Teaching Package for Occupational Health Services.* RCN Society of Occupational Health Nursing.

Salvage, J. (2000) Now wash your hands ... hand hygiene remains the single most important means of preventing hospital-acquired infection. *Nursing Times* 96(43): 22.

Suleyman, F. (2000) Addressing the problem of latex glove allergy. *Community Nurse* 6(3): 26, 28.

Taylor, M. and Campbell, C. (2000) Introduction to instruments. *Back to Basics Perioperative Practice and Principles*. Harrogate: NATN.

Williams, M.J., Clancy, J. and McVicar, A.J. (eds) (2001) How do you keep your patient safe? Biological issues that impact on procedure. *British Journal of Perioperative Nursing* 2(3): 124–30.

Woods, R.K. and Dellinger, E.P. (2000) Current guidelines for antibiotic prophylaxis of surgical wounds. *American Family Physician* 57(11): 19–28, 2731–40.

Answers to multiple choice questions

Q., p. 116

c   actively multiplying bacteria are present in the blood stream.

Q.1, p. 126

d   anticoagulant therapy.

Q.2, p. 126

c   reassure patient and place in a comfortable upright position.

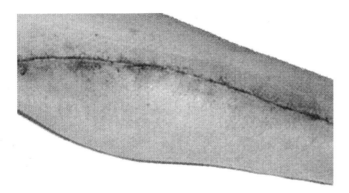

Plate 4i **Wound healing by primary intention or closure as occurs with, for example, surgical incision.** The wound is closed to eliminate the dead space and held together by sutures or clips. There is minimal granulation and a low risk of scarring; if scarring is present, it fades with time and disappears when wound healing is matured. Primary closure is not appropriate with infected or long-standing wounds

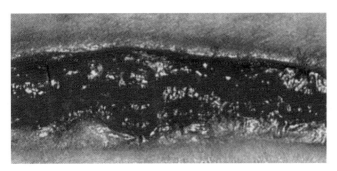

Plate 4ii **Wound healing by secondary intention or closure as occurs with, for example, leg ulceration where there is a lot of tissue lost or when there is a risk of infection.** The wound is left open to heal by granulation. Cosmetically the results are comparable to primary intention

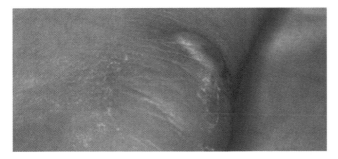

Plate 4iii **Wound showing the classical signs of inflammation**

Q. List the classical signs of inflammation.

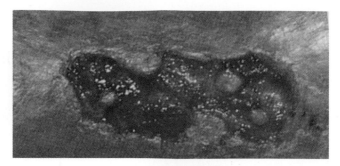

***Plate 4iv* Wound showing signs of healthy granulation.** Note that the wound has a bright red, moist and shiny appearance

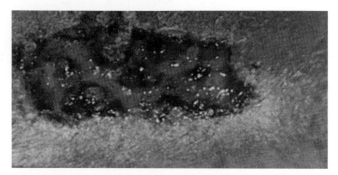

***Plate 4v* Wound showing signs of unhealthy granulation.** Note that the wound has a dark red colour (in parts) and a dehydrated and dull appearance

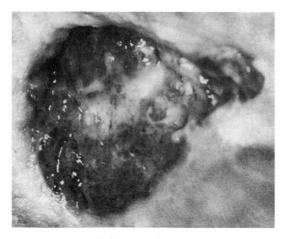

***Plate 4vi* Wound showing the process of epithelialization.** Note the pinkish-white skin around the edge of the wound

Chapter 5

Perioperative influences on cardiovascular homeostasis

Introduction: relation of the cardiovascular system to cellular homeostasis

Regardless of their clinical area, the time spent by nurses monitoring blood pressure, pulse rate and pulse strength serves to emphasize the importance of the cardiovascular system to health. The relation of this system to cellular homeostasis is that it delivers nutrients, oxygen, hormones, etc. to the cells of the body and removes 'waste' products of metabolism from them, so preventing toxicity. The system, therefore, provides the transport 'hardware' that keeps blood continuously circulating in order to fulfil intracellular requirements.

The flow of blood to specific tissues usually reflects the metabolic demands of that tissue and so must be responsive to changing needs. Blood flow can be compromised in various ways. Of particular relevance to the trauma of surgery are the potential effects on blood pressure of losing too much body fluid, and of anaesthetic agents that depress blood pressure control by the autonomic nervous system. The aim of this chapter is to highlight those processes that normally maintain a continuous circulation of blood, especially the homeostatic control of arterial blood pressure (Figure 5.1). A more extensive discussion is available in Clancy and McVicar (2002); this text will enable the reader to complete the learning activities included in this chapter.

Overview of the anatomy and physiology of the cardiovascular system

The heart

The main role of the heart is to promote unidirectional flow of blood throughout the body. As part of this role, the action of the heart is responsible for maintaining a sufficient arterial blood pressure sufficiently to provide an adequate blood supply to all tissues.

EXERCISE

Using an anatomy and physiology textbook, identify the location of the heart. At what point on the chest is the heartbeat most readily palpated?

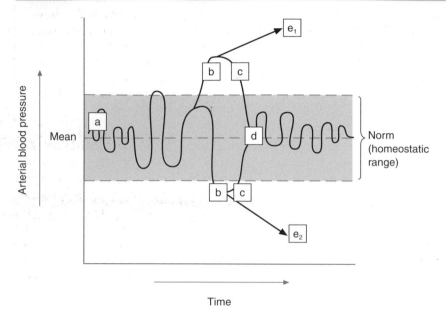

Figure 5.1 **A schematic illustration of the homeostatic regulation of arterial blood pressure**

a mean arterial blood pressure fluctuating within its homeostatic range.

b changes in arterial blood pressure as a consequence of altered cardiac function, changes in blood volume, or inappropriate changes in the distribution of blood to tissues.

c correction of the homeostatic imbalance. In the short and medium term, this normally entails changes in the activity of the autonomic nervous system, which alter cardiovascular parameters. In the long term, hormonal responses act to regulate the blood volume. In disordered states, therapies may include relaxation/stress coping mechanisms, or pharmacological methods to artificially alter cardiac function, blood volume or tissue blood flow (e.g. antihypertensive drugs when blood pressure is elevated).

d blood pressure homeostasis re-established.

e failure of homeostatic processes or interventions to correct the imbalance, for example in persistent hypertension (e1) or in shock (e2).

Figure 5.2 (opposite) ***a*** **A frontal section of the heart to show the main features and the direction of blood flow;** ***b*** **a normal electrocardiogram of a single heartbeat**

P, Q, R, S, T are the letters assigned to the deflections, or waves, from the baseline (see Figure 5.4)

Box 5.1   Application: access to the heart for open-heart surgery

During open-heart surgery the access to the heart is through the rib cage (Figure 5.3). The patient is placed in a supine position (Figure 1.1a) and a mid-sternum incision is made. Generally diathermy is used to cauterize (and hence seal) small bleeding vessels and to restrict blood loss and achieve haemostasis as well as for cutting through tissue. Once the sternum is in view, a finger is used to ensure that the xiphisternum is free, before a saw is placed in position. The sternum is then sawn symmetrically lengthways. Haemostasis (i.e. cessation of blood loss) from the split ends of bone is achieved by rubbing bone wax on the splintered parts. The ribs are retracted to expose the heart. During closure steel wires are used to hold the sternum together.

The heart operates as a double pump, since it has left and right sided functions that serve two distinctive circulatory circuits: the systemic circulation, and the pulmonary circulation, respectively. The interior of the heart is divided into two upper chambers called atria (atrium; singular), and two lower chambers called ventricles; each side of the heart is comprised of an atrium and a ventricle. The atria are the receiving chambers for blood returning from the circulation, via (on the right side) the inferior and superior vena cavae and the coronary sinus, and (on the left side) the pulmonary veins. The ventricles are the discharging chambers; the right ventricle ejects blood into the pulmonary 'trunk' artery, the left into the aorta. The path of blood flow through the heart chambers is illustrated in Figure 5.2a.

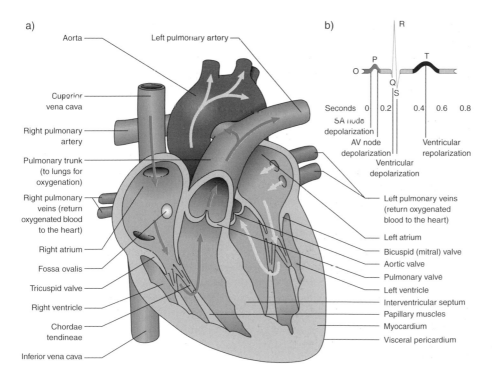

Box 5.2   Application: myocardial preservation during cardiac surgery and interoperative autotransfusion

During cardiac surgery ischaemic damage to the heart must be minimized and the myocardium preserved. In the past, for cardiac surgery to be performed it was necessary to immobilize the heart, empty the chambers and induce ventricular asystole. To achieve this, cooling of the heart using a cardioplegia solution and cardio-pulmonary bypass was used. Surgical advances and the development of Minimal Access Surgery have enabled cardiac surgeons to develop new techniques, which avoid using cardioplegia and cardio-pulmonary bypass. One recent development is minimal access coronary artery bypass grafting; the surgery is performed on the beating heart, thus avoiding the need to immobilize the heart. Advances in minimal access surgery mean that many cardiac procedures are now being performed in this way.

Autotransfusion or autologous blood transfusion describes the collection and donation of blood from and to the same patient. The two most common ways this can be achieved are, first, when the patient donates their own blood pre-operatively, and receives it later during surgery or during the post-operative period. Second, blood can be collected during the surgery and processed to return red cells to the patient during the perioperative period.

Intraoperative autotransfusion is when salvaged blood is sucked from the operative site using a sterile closed system through a filter containing a mixture of normal saline and heparin; this prevents the blood from clotting within the filter and the centrifuge system. Once there is sufficient blood loss (this varies depending on the system used), the blood can be processed. The blood is transferred into a centrifuge system where it is washed in normal saline. This process separates the non-cellular, cellular and biochemical debris from the red blood cells and eliminates 95–99 per cent of unwanted contamination. The debris might include bone or tissue fragments, fatty lipids, fatty acids, fibrinolytic factors and plasma. The salvaged red blood cells are transferred into a blood transfusion bag and then through a blood administration set back to the patient. Intraoperative autotransfusion is commonly used in major vascular surgery, for example aortic aneurysm repair, cardiac surgery, trauma and orthopaedic surgery, and in situations where there is an anticipated blood loss of greater than 20 per cent of the patient's blood volume. Contraindications to autotransfusion include presence of bowel contents, the presence of tumour cells, urine and some irrigating fluids.

EXERCISE

Consider the indications and contraindications to autotransfusion and suggest how they could affect the homeostatic controls within the body.

EXERCISE

Familiarize yourself with the chambers of the heart, their associated vessels and the structure and functions of the heart wall.

Box 5.3   Application: congenital heart defects, cardiac tamponade and pericarditis

Most congenital cardiac defects result from teratogenic influences during the early stages of pregnancy when the heart is developing. Such defects account for approximately one half of all infant deaths arising from congenital abnormalities. The most frequent are septal defects and a patent ductus arteriosus (i.e. a vessel between the pulmonary artery and aorta that allows most of the blood to bypass the lungs in the foetus). A failure of closure of the foramen ovale soon after birth results in an atrial septal defect (ASD); this is commonly referred to as a 'hole in the heart'.

Blood passes from the right side of the heart to the lungs for oxygenation; cardiac defects involving right-to-left shunts (e.g. Tetralogy of Fallot, transposition of the great vessels, i.e. the aorta and pulmonary arterial trunk) prevent complete oxygenation of blood. Significant defects cause cyanosis (a blue colouration of the skin and mucous membranes due to low oxygen content of blood). This may be initially treated with oxygen therapy depending upon the severity of the cyanosis, later with corrective surgical techniques to abolish the shunts and/or vessel abnormalities.

Corrective surgery for congenital heart defects often requires cardiopulmonary bypass; in neonates it is technically more difficult than in older children. Palliative surgery may be carried out in younger children and correction of the defect performed when the child is older. Surgery for atrial septal defects is performed through the right atrium; the defect can be sutured or patched. Tetralogy of Fallot may be treated palliatively at first and total correction undertaken before the child starts school. In children with poor pulmonary blood flow and severe cyanosis, a palliative shunt between the subclavian artery and pulmonary artery may be performed; this provides an increase in pulmonary blood flow and improved oxygenation. Corrective surgery involves closing the shunt, removing the outflow obstruction and closure of the ventricular septal defect.

Conditions comprising left-to-right shunts (e.g. patent ductus arteriosus, patent foramen ovale and ventricular septal defects) increase pulmonary blood flow and lead to congestive heart failure if not corrected; early surgery is always advised. If the child has cardiac failure with patent ductus arteriosus, urgent surgery is required.

Correction involves controlling the consequential pulmonary oedema, providing respiratory support and restricting fluids. If the imbalance does not correct itself Frusemide, a loop diuretic, may be prescribed in order to reduce blood volume and cardiac congestion, and again surgical closure may be necessary.

An excessive build-up of the pericardial fluid or extensive bleeding into the pericardium is potentially life threatening due to the consequential compression (called cardiac tamponade) of the heart tissue. This can stop the heart from beating. This excess fluid or blood needs to be removed (aspirated) to prevent this. The causes of tamponade are varied; an analysis of the aspirate aids a diagnosis. Aspiration alone may be enough, but corrective surgery may be required if the underlying cause is trauma, aneurysm or a complication of surgery.

Cardiac tamponade is corrected through a small anterior thoracotomy and the pressure released if the tamponade is caused by trauma to the heart (e.g. stab injury), there can be a dramatic improvement in the patient's condition once the pressure is released. However, the underlying cause must be managed to prevent the recurrence of the tamponade.

Both deficiency and excessive accumulation of pericardial fluid can lead to inflammation of the pericardium, a condition known as pericarditis. This is often associated with a painful 'pericardial friction rub' of the parietal and visceral membranes which can be heard on auscultation. Pericardial disease causes the formation of fibrous tissue around the heart, which prevents the heart from fully expanding. This in turn causes systemic venous congestion; surgery may become necessary. Surgical access to the heart is achieved through a vertical sternotomy and the fibrous tissue is dissected off the heart. This surgery can be performed with or without cardio-pulmonary bypass.

Cardiac cycle

Each heartbeat represents a relaxation/filling phase (called diastole), and a contraction/ejection phase (called systole), for the ventricles. The events, which occur during these phases in a single heartbeat, are called the cardiac cycle. The filling and emptying of chambers on the right and left sides of the heart occur simultaneously at the appropriate stage of the cycle, and so the actions of the two pumps are matched.

EXERCISE

Identify the location of the four heart valves illustrated in Figure 5.2a.

Box 5.4   Application: normal heart sounds and heart murmurs

When listening to the heart with a stethoscope, one does not hear the opening of the valves, as this is a silent, relatively slow process. Valve closure is more sudden, however, and the sudden pressure differentials that develop across the valve produce vibrations of the valve and the surrounding fluid. The sounds given off travel in all directions through the chest; these are best heard at the surface of the chest in locations that differ slightly from the actual location of the valves (see Figure 5.3). When ventricles first contract, the closure of the AV valves produces a long and booming sound since the vibration is low in pitch and is of relatively long duration. This is the first heart (or Korotkoff) sound and is described as 'lub'. The second heart sound – 'dup' – is caused by the closure of the semilunar valves at the beginning of ventricular relaxation. This sound is a relatively rapid 'snap' since valve closure is extremely fast, and thus the surroundings vibrate for a lesser period of time.

A heart murmur is an abnormal sound consisting of a rushing or gurgling noise that is heard before, between or after the normal heart sounds, or even masking the normal heart sounds. Most murmurs indicate a valve disorder. Certain infectious diseases of the endocardium can damage heart valves, because they are also endocardium.

Endocardial damage can be either congenital or acquired. Acquired damage causes inflammation, or ischaemia, degenerative or infectious alterations of valve structure and hence function. The usual cause of acquired valve dysfunction is inflammation of the endocardium; secondary to acute rheumatic fever (most sufferers are now elderly, having had rheumatic fever in childhood) this usually follows a streptococcal infection of the throat. These bacteria stimulate an immunological response in which antibodies attack these pathogens also causing inflammation of the connective tissue of the heart valves. This can cause the cusps of the valve to stick together, thus narrowing their opening (a process called stenosis). Subsequent damage to the edges of the cusps impairs closure and backward flow occurs. The valve is now said to be 'leaky' or incompetent. Although stenosis and incompetence may coexist, one often predominates.

In both instances the pumping efficiency of the heart declines and, as a consequence, the workload of the heart is increased. However, severe valve deformity is required to cause serious impairment, in these cases the heart ultimately becomes weakened, and this can cause heart failure. The mitral valve is usually affected since pressure differentials developed by the left ventricle are greater than those across the tricuspid valve in the right. Mitral incompetence and mitral stenosis occur in 10–15 per cent of the population. Valve dysfunction is treated with:

■ cardiac glycosides. The most commonly used cardiac glycoside is digoxin, which increases the force of myocardial contraction and reduces the oxygen consumption of the heart. Where there is severe heart failure such as in cardiogenic shock and hypoperfusion of the brain and kidneys, an intravenous infusion of dobutamine and dopamine may be given. Dobutamine increases heart contractility and stimulates the beta-1 adrenoceptors in the heart. Renal perfusion is increased with dopamine and there is also stimulation of the beta-1 adrenoceptors.

- diuretics. Loop diuretics, e.g. frusemide, inhibit sodium chloride (NaCl) reabsorption in the loop of Henle, where NaCl absorption is high. They are used for patients with pulmonary oedema caused by moderate to severe heart failure, and for reducing peripheral and pulmonary oedema. For patients with mild forms of heart failure and hypertension, bendrofluazide is commonly used; unlike loop diuretics it acts on the distal tubule of the kidney where there is less NaCl reabsorption, thus sparing potassium.
- dietary salt restriction. A low NaCl intake is associated with a reduction in blood volume (Chapter 3).
- antibiotics. Penicillin is the drug of choice in the prevention of endocarditis, for patients with heart valve defects or prosthetic valves. A broad-spectrum antibiotic such as amoxycillin is most commonly used, as it is active against gram-positive and gram-negative bacteria, as well as strains of Escherichia coli, Haemophilus influenza and Salmonella. For patients who are allergic to penicillin, a combination of vancomycin and gentamycin might be used (see pp. 93–4).

If, however, the mitral stenosis or the insufficiency is severe, the following surgical interventions may be required:

- open commissurotomy. This involves the separation of the fused leaflets of the stenosed valve, during open-heart surgery.
- mitral annuloplasty. This involves the reduction of a dilated annulus, which is contributing to back flow of blood. The reduction is achieved by sutures or by the insertion of a prosthetic ring.
- mitral valve replacement. During this procedure the mitral valve leaflets, chordae tendineae and papillary muscles are excised and replaced by a mechanical prosthesis.

(Heuther and McCance 1996)

Systolic and diastolic murmurs

A systolic murmur is one heard during systole, whilst diastolic murmurs are heard after the second heart sound.

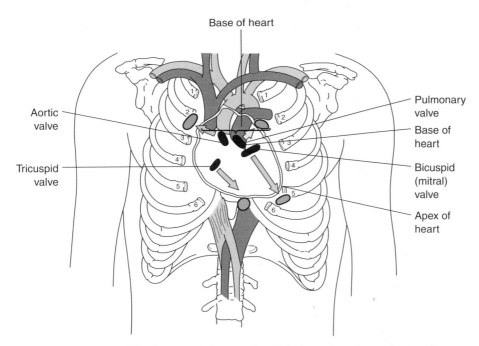

Base of heart

Aortic valve

Tricuspid valve

Pulmonary valve

Base of heart

Bicuspid (mitral) valve

Apex of heart

Figure 5.3 **Location of the heart and heart valves (black spot) and auscultation sites (blue spot) for heart sounds**
The heart is located within the mediastinum, which is the middle region of the thoracic cavity

Q. Describe the anatomical location of the stethoscope whereby mitral stenosis would be most audible.

The orderly and co-ordinated contraction of the heart chambers during the cardiac cycle is controlled by an intrinsic regulatory mechanism, involving the cardiac conduction system of specialized muscle tissue.

EXERCISE

Using a physiology textbook, identify the following components of the heart's conduction system: sinoatrial node, the atrioventricular node, the Bundles of His, and Purkinje fibres. Now draw their positions on Figure 5.2a.

The impulse, which will eventually cause the heart to contract, is initiated within the sinoatrial node located in the right atrium. The rate of heartbeat is largely determined by the intrinsic properties of the node, but is altered by the influence of the autonomic nervous system, or by blood-borne hormones such as thyroxine and adrenaline. The impulse spreads from the node and causes atrial contraction. It then arrives at the atrioventricular (AV) node, which distributes it to the ventricles via the Bundles of His and Purkinje fibres. The slower conducting properties of the AV node allow the atria time to empty their blood into the ventricles, before the ventricles begin their contraction.

The electrocardiogram (ECG) reflects the electrical changes associated with muscle contraction (Figure 5.2b). The ECG is therefore useful in diagnosing abnormal cardiac rhythms, cardiac pathology and in following the course of recovery from myocardial damage. Its ease of measurement also makes it useful as an aid to monitor cardiac activity during, for example, surgical procedures. The ECG is used during anaesthesia to monitor cardiac function, providing early indications of rhythm disturbances, problems with the anaesthesia or, for example, when surgery is being performed close to the heart, causing cardiac disturbances.

Box 5.5   Application: ectopic beats

Stimulants such as caffeine and nicotine, when used in excessive amounts, may increase the excitability of heart muscle to such a degree that ectopic beats result in abnormal contractions. Other triggers of ectopics are electrolyte imbalances, hypoxia and toxic reactions to drugs, such as digitalis (see Figure 5.4c–e).

EXERCISE

Using your reader, identify the major vessels that comprise the coronary circulation.

Figure 5.4 (opposite) **Cardiac arrthymias**

Q. Refer to Figure 5.2b to describe what the wave and interval components of the ECG represent and what is meant by the term sinus rhythm.

a   Sinus tachycardia. The heart rate at rest >100 beats/min.

Q. Identify the conditions that cause sinus tachycardia.

b   Sinus bradycardia. The heart rate at rest is <60 beats/min.

Q. What is the treatment for this arrhythmia?

c   Atrial flutter. The characteristic atrial 'saw tooth' waves appear at a regular interval and at a rate between 250–400.

Q. How many atrial impulses reach the ventricles?

d   Atrial fibrillation (AF). Atrial waves are rapid, small and irregular waves

Q. Using your reader, list three causes of AF.

e   Ventricular fibrillation (VF). Ventricular rhythm is rapid and chaotic

Q. Identify the treatment for a patient with VF.

f   Asystole. Ventricular standstill

Q. Identify two causes of asystole and treatment required.

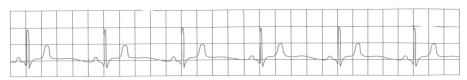

Normal sinus rhythm (included for reference)

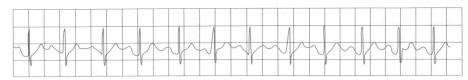

a)

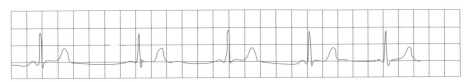

b)

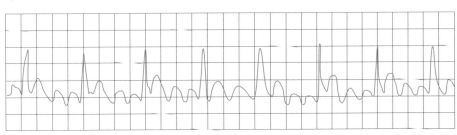

c)

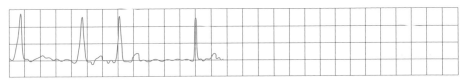

d)

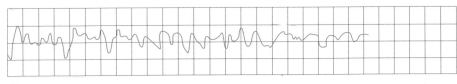

e)

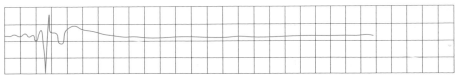

f)

Blood vessels

Blood is transported throughout the body via a network of specialized vessels:

- arteries and arterioles (i.e. smallest arteries) transport blood away from the heart,
- capillaries (and sinusoids in some tissues, e.g. the liver) exchange materials between blood, tissue fluid and cells,
- venules (i.e. smallest veins) and veins return blood to the heart (Figure 5.5).

EXERCISES

Using a physiology textbook:

1 identify the structure and composition of the walls of arteries and veins. How are they similar? How do they differ?
2 identify which forces (i.e. pressures) determine the exchange of water and nutrients between blood and tissue fluid across the walls of capillaries.
3 which substances in blood do not pass into the tissue fluid?

The walls of most blood vessels have three distinctive layers, or tunicae. The relative thickness and composition of each coat varies according to the functions of the vessel. For example, the tunica media (middle coat) of major arteries is relatively thick and contains considerable numbers of elastic fibres. These fibres facilitate stretching of the vessel to accommodate the extra blood volume and pressure instigated by ventricular contraction, promoting elastic recoil when blood ejection from the heart momentarily ceases during ventricular relaxation. Consequently, blood flows continuously around the body during the entire cardiac cycle.

The major arteries give rise to smaller but relatively more muscular arteries sometimes referred to as 'distributing arteries' because they distribute blood to peripheral tissues. Arterioles deliver blood to the capillary vessels within tissues. The diameter of arterioles, and the muscle tone of small sphincters where blood enters capillaries (called pre-capillary sphincters), are controlled both intrinsically, in response to changes in tissue fluid composition (a process called autoregulation), and extrinsically, by sympathetic nerves and certain hormones. Thus, the flow of blood into capillaries is regulated and can be altered according to the metabolic requirements of cells within the specific capillary networks.

The venous system takes blood from capillary beds and returns it to the heart. En route, the vessels increase their diameter, their walls thicken, and they progress from the venules to the largest veins (the vena cavae). The lumens of veins are large for a given external diameter; they offer little resistance to blood flow, which is important because the pressure of blood within the venous circulation is low and provides little force to circulate blood. About two-thirds of the total blood volume is found within the venous system at any time, and this is why veins are referred to as the capacitance vessels or blood reservoirs. Their diameter, and hence capacity, is especially influenced by the level of activity of the sympathetic nervous system.

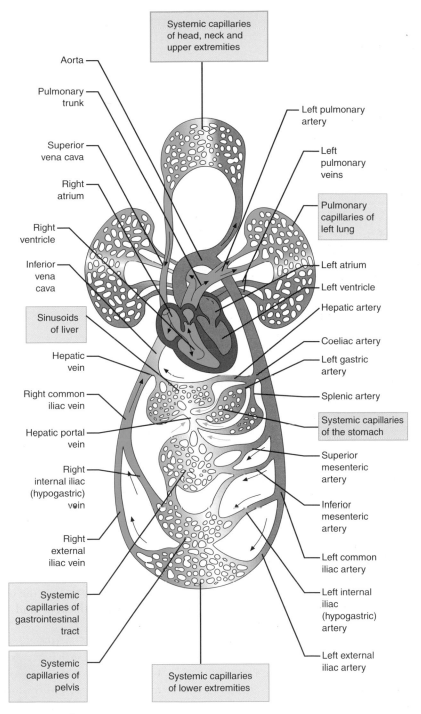

Aorta

Pulmonary trunk

Superior vena cava

Right atrium

Right ventricle

Inferior vena cava

Sinusoids of liver

Hepatic vein

Right common iliac vein

Hepatic portal vein

Right internal iliac (hypogastric) vein

Right external iliac vein

Systemic capillaries of gastrointestinal tract

Systemic capillaries of pelvis

Systemic capillaries of head, neck and upper extremities

Left pulmonary artery

Left pulmonary veins

Pulmonary capillaries of left lung

Left atrium

Left ventricle

Hepatic artery

Coeliac artery

Left gastric artery

Splenic artery

Systemic capillaries of the stomach

Superior mesenteric artery

Inferior mesenteric artery

Left common iliac artery

Left internal iliac (hypogastric) artery

Left external iliac artery

Systemic capillaries of lower extremities

Figure 5.5 **Circulatory routes**
Oxygenated blood is shown in grey, deoxygenated in dark blue

Box 5.6   Application: coronary arterial disease (CAD)

Ischaemic heart disease is the term used to describe a homeostatic imbalance that reflects myocardial oxygen insufficiency, arising from a narrowed or occluded coronary artery. Some individuals have no signs or symptoms ('silent' myocardial ischaemia); others experience angina pectoris (chest pain) or suffer a heart attack (myocardial infarction). Atherosclerotic plaques may cause the narrowing and be sufficient to cause the occlusion alone, or the plaques may become complicated by a blood clot formation causing the narrowing. If the narrowing progresses slowly, a collateral (alternative) arterial supply grows, effectively acting as a homeostatic control to replace the malfunctioned vessel. If, however, a sudden severe narrowing or occlusion occurs, the collateral circulation has insufficient time to develop, and consequently myocardial infarction may occur.

Angina pectoris literally means 'choked chest'. It may result from a variety of causes:

1   increased physical demands on the heart that cannot be met by the coronary circulation.
2   stress-induced spasms of the coronary arteries.
3   hypertension (which excessively increases the oxygen demands of the heart).
4   fever, which elevates cardiac activity and hence its oxygen needs.
5   hyperthyroidism (i.e. excessive release of thyroid hormones), which also increases cardiac activity.
6   aortic stenosis.
7   atherosclerosis.

A myocardial infarction, or coronary, occurs when the coronary arteries become completely occluded, cutting off blood flow to the tissue beyond the occlusion, resulting in the death of the myocardial tissue. A thrombus or embolus (i.e. a homeostatic failure of the clotting process) may cause occlusion in one of the coronary arteries. The after-effects depend partly on the size and location of the area of necrosis. In chronic ischaemic heart disease, small infarcts may give rise to myocardial weakness, angina, 'silent' myocardial infarction and heart failure. If the ischaemic heart disease is acute, then one or more large arteries are occluded and the atheroma is usually complicated by thrombosis. Consequently, a large infarct results, and death may occur as a result of acute heart failure, ventricular fibrillation (see Figure 5.4e), rupture of the ventricular wall, or pulmonary or cerebral embolism (leading to respiratory or cerebral failure).

Risk factors

Risk factors associated with CAD can be:

- modified with dietary alteration. For example, in conditions with a direct link to CAD, such as diabetes mellitus. People who are over-weight can reduce weight; those with high cholesterol may reduce their blood cholesterol levels.
- modified by changing other lifestyle habits. For example, cessation of smoking, changing type A (i.e. 'coronary') personality behaviours and adopting a moderate exercise programme, which actually reverse the process of CAD.
- controlled by medication. For example, anti-hypertensive therapy.
- not modified (i.e. beyond our control). These factors include genetic pre-disposition, age and gender. Adult males are more likely than adult females to develop CAD; after the age of seventy, their risks are roughly equal. The nurse role in health education and health promotion regarding minimizing the modifiable risk factors associated with individual patients is therefore vital as a preventative measure but also in minimizing the re-occurrence of CAD.

Diagnosis of CAD

Laboratory tests, haemodynamic tests, graphic investigations and radiological assessments are performed to assess the functioning of the heart and the coronary circulation (see Table 5.1).

The reader is advised to complete the exercises listed in Table 5.1 since the following only refers to cardiac catheterization and coronary angiocar-diography. This is an invasive procedure used to visualize the coronary arteries and assess the degree of the coronary occlusion. It is also used:

- to measure pressures in the chambers of the heart and blood vessels,
- to assess cardiac output (i.e. the quantity of blood ejected by the left ventricle each minute) and diastolic properties of the left ventricle,
- to measure the flow of blood through the heart and blood vessels, and the oxygen content of the blood,
- to assess the status of heart valves and conduction system,
- to identify the exact location of septal and valve defects,
- to inject clot-dissolving drugs (e.g. streptokinase) into the coronary arteries to dissolve an obstructing thrombus.

The procedure involves inserting a long flexible radiopaque cardiac catheter into a peripheral vein (for right heart catheterization) or peripheral artery (for left heart catheterization) guiding it under x-ray observance. A radiopaque dye is then injected into blood vessels or heart chambers.

Treatment of CAD

Failure of myocardial homeostasis thus requires clinical intervention to re-establish it. The angina patient, for example, is given vasodilator drugs (e.g. glyceryl trinitrate) to increase coronary flow or beta-blockers (e.g. Propanalol, atenolol and labetalol hydrochloride) to reduce myocardial oxygen requirements. The patient who has had an infarction may be given cholesterol-lowering drugs (e.g. Colestipol hydrochloride, bezafibrate and simvastatin) and/or clot-dissolving agents (e.g. streptokinase, alteplase and reteplase). Alternatively the patient may require a coronary bypass operation to remedy cardiac integrity, i.e. if a large area of the myocardium is affected and/or major vessels are occluded.

Coronary arterial by-pass grafting

This is a surgical procedure in which the patient's own long saphenous vein or internal mammary artery is used for the graft. The vein is removed at the same time as the bypass surgery and grafted on to the aorta and coronary arteries to bypass the area of obstruction. The grafted blood vessel is sutured between the aorta and the unblocked portion of the coronary artery.

Percutaneous transluminal coronary angioplasty (PTCA)

This non-surgical procedure involves a balloon catheter insertion into an artery of an arm or leg from where it is guided into a coronary artery. The angiograms are recorded to locate fatty plaques, the catheter is advanced to the point of obstruction and a balloon-like device is inflated with air to squash the plaque against the vessel wall. A special device resembling a spring coil (called a 'stent') is permanently placed in an artery to keep the artery patent (i.e. open), permitting blood to circulate. This is inserted in order to prevent the reoccurrence of the stenosis in the dilated arteries.

Cardiac output, peripheral resistance and blood pressure

Control of the circulation ensures that cellular homeostasis is not compromised by lack of resources or accumulation of excess substances. Factors that are instrumental in that control are:

1   the provision of adequate blood (via the cardiac output),
2   the regulation of the diameter of blood vessels (i.e. vascular resistance),
3   the provision of an adequate pressure gradient which favours blood flow through the tissues.

It is convenient to consider each factor individually but it is important to note their interactions, especially in relation to the control of arterial blood pressure.

Table 5.1 Investigations of cardiac function and coronary circulation

Laboratory tests	*Haemodynamic tests*
• Complete blood cell count • Serum: cardiac enzymes, lipids, electrolytes • Blood: urea nitrogen, glucose and coagulation tests • Urinalysis	• Central venous pressure • Pulmonary artery pressure • Cardiac output measurements • Intra-arterial pressure monitoring

ACTIVITIES

1 Explain the functional significance of the blood and urine tests used to investigate cardiac function.
2 List the cardiac specific enzymes used as an aid to diagnose myocardial infarction.

ACTIVITIES

1 How is haemodynamic monitoring carried out?
2 Explain how you can ensure patient safety during this type of monitoring.
3 Make notes on the procedures associated with each of the above tests not mentioned in this chapter.

Graphic investigations	*Radiological techniques*
• Electrocardiogram. This records the electrical activity of the heart • Echocardiography. Ultrasound is used to detect structural and functional changes • Scanning of the heart	Cardiac catheterization. A process to view the heart, the valves and circulation angiography. A process to view the status of the coronary circulation. • Myocardial perfusion imaging. A process to identify ischaemic tissue. • Myocardial infarct imaging. A process to identify the infarcted area.

ACTIVITIES

1 Identify the ECG changes that aid a diagnosis of a myocardial infarction.
2 Identify the echocardiography findings in a patient with severe mitral stenosis. Ask colleagues at work if you are having difficulty.

ACTIVITIES

1 Using the information detailed in Box 5.6 identify the procedure of cardiac catheterization and coronary angiocardiography.
2 How do you prepare a patient for the procedure?
3 What is the post-operative care given to the patient following this procedure?

Cardiac output

Cardiac output is the quantity of blood ejected by the left ventricle each minute. It is calculated by multiplying the stroke volume (volume ejected per contraction) by the number of heartbeats (ventricular contractions) per minute:

$$\text{Cardiac output} = \text{Stroke volume} \times \text{Heart rate}$$

The average heart rate at rest is 70 beats per minute, the stroke volume is 70 ml per beat, and so the cardiac output approximates to 5 litres per minute. Since the average adult blood volume is about 5 litres, this means that the entire blood volume passes through the heart every minute at rest. Cardiac output varies with the changing metabolic demands of the body, for example during exercise, where it rises when the heart rate and/or stroke volume increases.

EXERCISE

Identify the autonomic nerves which supply the heart and their origin in the brain stem. Which nerve increases cardiac activity and which decreases it?

Stroke volume represents the difference between the amount of blood that collects in a ventricle during diastole (called the end-diastolic volume, which is about 120 ml), and the amount of blood remaining in the ventricle after ventricular systole (called the end-systolic volume, which is about 50 ml at rest). The resting stroke volume, therefore, approximates to 70 ml. A change in either the end-diastolic or end-systolic volume will alter the stroke volume.

The end-diastolic volume (i.e. at the end of the filling phase) depends upon the venous return to the heart, and upon the time available for the ventricles to fill (which depends upon the heart rate). The end-systolic volume can be altered independently of the end-diastolic volume by changes in the contractility of the heart, since a more powerful contraction will empty the ventricles more efficiently. Sympathetic activity from the cardiac centre of the brain stem has this effect, as does adrenaline.

EXERCISE

Describe Starling's Law of the Heart.

Autonomic nerve stimulation, and some hormones, especially adrenaline, induce variations in the heart rate. The resting heart rate may also be influenced by drugs, which interfere with the neural control (e.g. anaesthetic agents, or sympathetic agonists and antagonists, see Box 5.11), and also by the presence of hypo- or hyperthermia.

> **Box 5.7   Application: clinical assessment of the cardiac output**
>
> Cardiac output can be assessed by direct or indirect means. Indirect methods may include measuring related variables, such as the urinary output, or peripheral tone and limb temperatures. These variables are used to classify the cardiac output as being high, normal or low. However, a more accurate, direct and repeatable measurement such as thermodilution is required to monitor treatment in critically ill patients. Thermodilution involves inserting a triple lumen Swan–Ganz catheter, with a thermistor (temperature sensor) located at its tip, into a peripheral vein and advancing it to the right atrium. Subsequently, a bolus of cold saline of a known temperature is injected into the catheter. As the saline and right atrial blood mix, the temperature changes and this is sensed by a thermistor placed in the arterial system, which records when the bolus passes its tip. The actual temperature recorded will depend upon the time taken for the bolus to reach this thermistor and the volume of blood into which the cold saline was dispersed. The data obtained can be used to calculate the cardiac output. Recent technology has largely superseded this method by using imaging techniques to assess cardiac output. This methodology is non-invasive and also provides moment-to-moment evaluation of changes.

Peripheral resistance

Changes in the diameter of blood vessels provide the main means of varying the resistance to flow provided by blood vessels: the smaller the diameter, the greater the resistance to blood flow. Even small changes in the diameter of a vessel will have a significant effect on the conduction of blood through it.

If blood supply is inadequate and tissues become deficient in oxygen (i.e. ischaemic), cells respond by releasing carbon dioxide, lactic acid and other metabolites, and these substances are responsible for causing local arterioles and precapillary sphincters to relax, thus increasing blood flow and oxygen availability. Tissues, therefore, are capable of autoregulating their own blood supply independently of extrinsic influences. This intrinsic mechanism helps to regulate tissue blood supply at rest and is also important for meeting changed nutritional demands, like that occurring in muscle during exercise.

The diameter of arterioles is also influenced by neural and hormonal mechanisms. In particular, the diameter is regulated by sympathetic nerve activity from the vasomotor centre of the brain stem. The normal background level of activity sets the basal muscle tone of arterioles throughout the body, determining the total resistance of the entire circulation (called the total peripheral resistance). Thus, changes in sympathetic output can cause either vasoconstriction or dilation and so increase or decrease the peripheral resistance, respectively. In reality, changes in sympathetic activity influence individual tissues to varying degrees; for example, the circulation through the brain is little affected. Under some circumstances there is also selective change; for example the change in skin blood flow in relation to body temperature control.

> **EXERCISE**
>
> Arterioles provide the main means of varying resistance to blood flow through tissues. Identify three other factors that also influence how easily blood flows through a vessel.

Blood pressure

The flow rate of any fluid is proportional to the pressure applied to that fluid. Thus fluid flows from high to low pressure regions and the greater the pressure differential, the faster the movement. Blood circulates because the heart pump establishes a pressure gradient.

The systemic arterial pressure in resting young adult moves between about 120 and 80 mmHg (millimetres of mercury) during a single cardiac cycle. The higher value is observed following ejection of blood from the left ventricle during systole and so is called the systolic pressure. The lower value is that observed at the end of diastole and so is called the diastolic pressure. The difference between the two is called the pulse pressure and provides information about the condition of blood vessels and also about the stroke volume.

> **EXERCISE**
>
> Kilopascals (kPa) are SI units of blood pressures that will eventually replace millimetres of mercury mmHg. The conversion rate is 1 kPa = 7.6 mmHg).
>
> Calculate in kPa the systolic and diastolic blood pressure in a resting young adult.

Box 5.8   Application: thready and bounding pulses

A pulse that is weak and difficult to feel is often described as 'thready'. A thready pulse will usually be rapid and may be obliterated by pressure on the artery suggesting that the patient is dehydrated, bleeding or exhausted. In such cases, it may be necessary to feel the carotid or femoral pulse. Cardiac arrest should not be diagnosed simply because a radial pulse cannot be felt. In contrast, infection, stress, anaemia or exercise can result in a very strong and 'bounding' pulse.

Other variations in pulse, and their possible causes, are listed below.

- an irregularity that occurs regularly might be a cyclical event that could be the result of a heart block.
- an irregular rhythm is often the result of atrial fibrillation, which is the most common irregularity of cardiac rhythm occurring in 2–4 per cent of the adult population aged sixty plus.
- an occasional irregularity may be perceived as a 'missed' or 'dropped' beat. Often the result of occasional and ventricular ectopics (an 'extra beat' followed by a compensatory pause) which should be reported but might not be treated; healthy people report occasional ectopics.

The highest average blood pressure is observed in the aortic arch before the branches forming the coronary arteries, where it approximates to 95 mmHg (= 12.5 kPa); the lowest is where the vena cavae enter the right atrium, where it approximates to 3–5 mmHg (= 0.39–0.66 kPa). The relatively small pressures of the venous system means that arterial pressure approximates to the circulatory pressure gradient.

Box 5.9   Application: central venous pressure (CVP)

Although observation of the jugular vein in the neck gives a crude indication of the venous pressure (for example, a raised jugular venous pressure (JVP) may indicate cardiac failure) it is the central venous pressure (CVP) which is the most frequently monitored venous pressure. This is the pressure in the central veins (the superior and inferior vena cavae) as they enter the heart. As the tip of the catheter used to measure CVP lies in the right atrium, CVP is equivalent to right atrial pressure (CVP is measured in CmH_2O because of its low pressures). The catheter is radiopaque and its position is confirmed by a chest x-ray. If the tricuspid valve is normal, the CVP equals the end diastolic pressure in the right ventricle and therefore is an index of right ventricular function. Impaired right ventricular function would lead to a back pressure that would raise the pressure in the atrium and hence give a higher CVP reading.

   The volume of blood returning to the heart (venous return) is the other major determinant of the CVP. Changes in circulatory fluid volume and the venomotor tone will alter the venous return: an increase in a circulatory fluid volume or venomotor tone will increase the venous return and give a higher CVP reading and vice versa. The major clinical advantages of CVP measurement is that it monitors the circulating blood volume; it is used to manage fluid replacement therapy in hypovolaemia that may occur following burns, haemorrhage or surgery. Sequential measurements give an indication of adequate fluid replacement therapy and also help to prevent fluid overload.

Blood pressure homeostasis: responses to haemorrhage

The two principal factors that influence arterial blood pressure are the cardiac output and the peripheral resistance. The factors are related by the equation:

$$\text{Blood pressure} = \text{cardiac output} \times \text{total peripheral resistance.}$$

It is clear from the earlier discussion that sympathetic nerves and certain hormones are central to the control of these parameters. Collectively, their actions regulate the arterial blood pressure, especially when the circulation is compromised either in health (e.g. postural changes, exercise) or in ill-health (e.g. during haemorrhage).

Neural mechanisms provide immediate responses to haemorrhage (see Figure 5.6). Thus, reductions in cardiac output as a consequence of a decreased blood volume promote a decrease in blood pressure, and this is detected by stretch receptors (called baroreceptors) located within the circulatory system, primarily in the aortic arch and carotid arteries. Information from these receptors is conducted to the brain stem, and resultant sympathetic activity from the cardiovascular control centres has *three* main actions:

1   promoting vasoconstriction of arterioles in tissues, not in the heart and brain, and hence an increase in peripheral resistance.
2   increasing heart rate and ventricular contractility; these are mechanisms which act to restore cardiac output, although the reduced venous return due to blood loss often means that cardiac output remains depressed in spite of these actions. The increased heart rate in response to sympathetic stimulation, and the decreased pulse pressure as a consequence of a reduced stroke volume, is readily detected by palpation.
3   promoting venous constriction, and the release of blood from the spleen, contributing to an increase in the volume of blood within the arteries.

Box 5.10   Application: 'carotid sinus syncope' and 'carotid sinus massage'

Because of the anatomical position of the carotid sinus (i.e. close to the anterior surface of the neck), it is possible to stimulate the baroreceptors by applying external pressure on this region of the neck. Anything that stretches or applies pressure to the carotid sinus (such as hyperextension of the head, tight collars or carrying heavy shoulder loads) may slow the heart rate and cause 'carotid sinus syncope'. That is, fainting due to inappropriate stimulation of the carotid sinus baroreceptors.

Physicians sometimes use 'carotid sinus massage' to manipulate cardiac function. This involves carefully massaging the neck over the carotid sinus, to slow the heart rate. Such a technique is useful in a patient who has paroxysmal supraventricular tachycardia, a type of tachycardia that originates in the atria.

In patients who have chronic hypertension (chronic = persisting for some years), the baroreceptors seem to be reset to maintain pressure at a higher set point.

The control of blood pressure is highly effective and even a 20 per cent reduction in blood volume may not produce a decrease in blood pressure, although intense vasoconstriction may eventually compromise tissue functioning and promote shock. The excessive stimulation of sympathetic activity as part of the 'alarm' response to trauma may even promote an increase in blood pressure when body fluid losses are more moderate (Chapter 7).

Haemorrhage is usually also accompanied by the release of various hormones including adrenaline, angiotensin II, aldosterone, antidiuretic hormone and erythropoietin (Figure 5.6). Some of these influence peripheral resistance, but

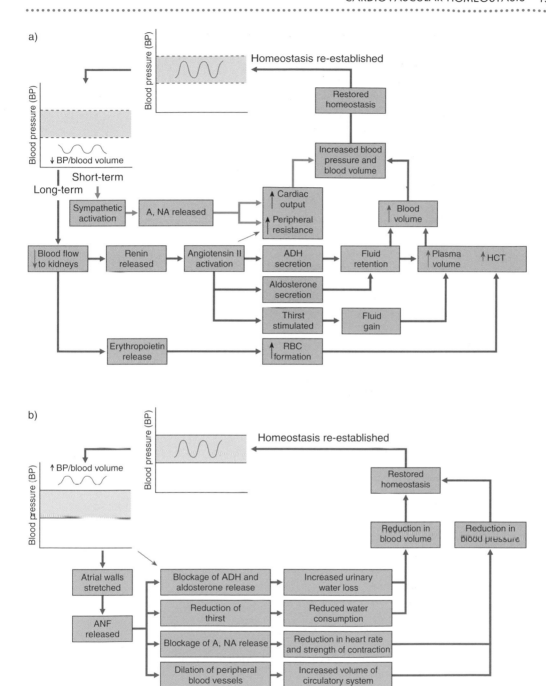

Figure 5.6 **Short- and long-term responses in the homeostatic regulation of arterial blood pressure following haemorrhage**
A, adrenaline; NA, noradrenaline; ADH, antidiuretic hormone; HCT, haematocrit; atrial antiuretic factor ANF, ↑ increased; ↓ decreased

hormonal actions also include modulating the renal excretion of electrolytes and water, and influencing red blood cell synthesis; that is, they are regulators of blood volume. Such hormones are considered to be medium or long-term regulators of blood pressure.

EXERCISES

1 This section has identified a number of hormones that are released following haemorrhage. Find out where in the body they are produced.

2 Which of the following is correct?

An arterial haemorrhage can be recognized from the fact that the blood normally
  a spurts from the proximal side of the wound.
  b spurts from the distal side of the wound.
  c wells up evenly from the proximal side of the wound.
  d wells up evenly from the distal side of the wound.

3 Haemorrhage is suspected when:
  a the temperature of the patient's body rises.
  b the pulse rate increases and the blood pressure falls.
  c the pulse rate falls and the blood pressure rises.
  d pulse rate drops and the respiratory rate rises.

See the end of this chapter for the answers to questions 2 and 3.

Box 5.11   Application: overview of pharmacology associated with cardiovascular homeostasis

It is common for cardiac dysrhythmias and hypotension to occur under anaesthesia. Anaesthetic agents can produce depression of the heart and of the motor tone of the peripheral vessels (Chapter 7). The homeostatic control mechanisms mentioned above (pp. 157–60) are largely responsible for the maintenance of normal blood pressure in a fit person during surgery. However, in cases where deeper anaesthesia is used or in the elderly or people with other predisposing problems, these mechanisms may be unable to regulate the blood pressure within the normal homeostatic range. Drug therapy then becomes necessary to regulate the blood pressure.

Adrenoceptor agonists

Adrenaline (also known as epinephrine) acts on both the alpha and beta adrenoceptors in the sympathetic nervous system. Alpha actions cause coronary and peripheral vasoconstriction, whilst the beta action causes an increase in heart rate, increased myocardial contractility and coronary vasodilation. Adrenaline is used in cardiac arrest to stimulate the heart without causing peripheral vasodilation and a resulting fall in blood pressure. It is used to preserve coronary and cerebral blood flow.

Isoprenaline works by selectively stimulating the beta-receptors. It causes the rate and force of the heartbeat to increase (thus increasing myocardial oxygen demand). It also relaxes smooth muscle causing vasodilation. The diastolic and mean arterial pressures fall, leaving the systolic pressure relatively unchanged.

Dopamine, when given by intravenous infusion, stimulates the cardiac beta 1 adrenoceptors. It is also given in low doses to increase renal perfusion, causing selective renal vasoconstriction and an increase in the blood pressure, ultimately increasing urine production. The dose is critical; a high dose can induce vasoconstriction and exacerbate heart failure. It is therefore important that it is used when invasive haemodynamic monitoring of the patient is in place.

Ephedrine raises the blood pressure by increasing the heart rate and myocardial contractility and promoting peripheral vasoconstriction. It is a synthetic drug, which is chemically related to adrenaline, although its effects last much longer.

Alpha adrenoceptor blocking drugs

These drugs reduce arteriolar and venous tone, causing a fall in peripheral resistance, hypotension and a fall in central venous pressure. These blockers reverse the effects of adrenaline and noradrenaline causing a fall in peripheral resistance. Extra intravenous fluids need to be given to maintain the circulation following administration of these drugs.

Phentolamine is used in a number if different ways. It promotes vasodilation in cardio-pulmonary bypass surgery, it antagonizes vasoconstriction in situations such as cardiogenic shock, it also acts as a myocardial stimulant by blocking the actions of adrenaline and noradrenaline on peripheral vessels causing vasodilation. There is a resulting fall in blood pressure and central venous pressure; therefore, extra intravenous fluid is required to maintain circulation

Beta adrenoceptor blocking drugs

Beta adrenoceptor blocking drugs all competitively block the beta 1–receptors. These drugs have varying lipid solubility and cardio-selectivity and are effective in reducing blood pressure and angina.

Atenolol is usually the drug of choice for prophalaxis of angina. It is a cardioselective beta blocking drug and acts by slowing the heart rate and reducing the myocardial demand for oxygen. It is effective in the treatment of cardiac dysrhythmias and hypertension.

Propanalol acts by antagonizing the beta 1 and beta 2 effects of isoprenaline on the heart and bronchi. There is a fall in heart rate and cardiac output and myocardial oxygen consumption is reduced. Propanalol is used to effectively control ectopic heartbeats, having a more effective response on atrial ectopics; it is also useful when treating arrhythmias caused by an overdose of digitalis. It is useful in controlling supraventricular tachycardia, tachycardia resulting from the use of hypotensive drugs, and excess adrenaline, and to reduce myocardial oxygen consumption, thus reducing the incidence of angina.

Other beta adrenoceptor blocking drugs (such as *Oxprenolol* and *Atenolol*) slow the heart rate and reduce myocardial oxygen demand. They are effective in the treatment of cardiac dysrhythmias and hypertension.

Labetalol is both an alpha and beta adrenoceptor blocker. It is useful in reducing myocardial oxygen consumption and in causing peripheral vasodilation. Because the alpha blocking effects are milder and of a shorter duration, the effects of the drug are similar to beta 1–adrenoceptor blocking drugs. It is commonly used during elective surgery to create a moderate reduction in blood pressure (Neal 1997).

EXERCISES

Drugs have chronotrophic and inotropic actions on the heart.

1 What do these terms mean?

2 Using the information in Box 5.11 (and your *British National Formulary* if you are experiencing difficulty) identify from the list below which drugs and bodily states have:
   a a positive inotropic action on the heart.
   b a positive chronotrophic action on the heart.
   c a negative inotropic action on the heart.
   d a negative chronotrophic action on the heart.

   ■ halothane (an anaesthetic)
   ■ isoprenaline
   ■ hyperkalaemia
   ■ adrenaline
   ■ Digoxin
   ■ Atropine
   ■ anoxia
   ■ digitalis
   ■ acidosis
   ■ Propananol.

Drugs that cause vasoconstriction and mimic the action of the sympathetic nervous system are called sympathomimetics.

3 Identify from the list above a drug that can be classed as sympathomimetic. Vasodilator drugs (i.e. adrenergic blockers) inhibit the activity of catecholamines at smooth muscle receptor sites and are used in the treatment of peripheral vascular decrease in order to increase blood flow to ischaemic tissues. These drugs increase blood flow to the skin rather than to the muscles, and are sometimes used in the treatment of varicose ulcers.

4 Identify a drug that operates in this way.
   Drugs can also directly effect the smooth muscle in the blood vessel wall, causing a relaxation, vasodilation.

5 Identify the potent vasodilator drug that is particularly effective in the treatment of angina.

Shock: a failure to maintain cardiovascular homeostasis

Introduction: shock and cellular homeostasis

A number of intricate processes are involved in the regulation of the cardiovascular system, all of which contribute to the maintenance of adequate oxygenation of tissues throughout the body, and the removal of the waste products of metabolism. The delivery of oxygen to cells by blood is vital because of their need to produce energy for the biochemical processes occurring within them; maintaining blood flow is therefore an essential contributor to cellular homeostasis (Figure 5.7).

The generation of energy by cells is measured by the yield of an intermediary substance, adenosine triphosphate (ATP); a single molecule of glucose will normally yield a net thirty-eight molecules of ATP. Biochemical processes, which require the presence of oxygen (that is, aerobically), produce thirty molecules of ATP; only eight ATP molecules are produced in the absence of oxygen (anaerobically). Thus, the production of ATP by a cell will be considerably compromised if the supply of oxygen to cells is insufficient. A further consequence of reduced aerobic metabolism is that less heat will be generated, since a larger amount of the energy released by respiration is liberated as heat. Anaerobic metabolism will therefore be a less efficient contributor to the regulation of body temperature. In addition, anaerobic metabolism produces lactic acid, which is potentially lethal to cells in high enough concentrations. Lactic acid must be removed from the tissues by blood; it is subsequently broken down in the liver by a process which also requires oxygen. The presence of excess lactic acid in a tissue causes pain, for example cramp pain in exercising muscle. Anaerobic respiration, therefore, is of limited use to the tissues.

EXERCISE

Find the relevant sections on aerobic and anaerobic metabolism in a physiology textbook (e.g. Clancy and McVicar 2002) and identify where in a cell oxygen is utilized to make ATP. What are the end products of the aerobic metabolism of glucose?

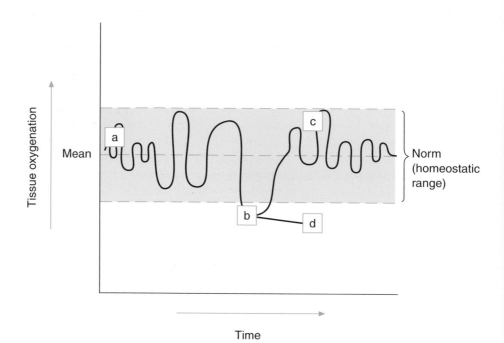

Figure 5.7 **Tissue oxygenation as a homeostatic process**

a Homeostatis – when oxygen supply to the cell is sufficient for cellular biochemical activities (metabolism).

b Falling oxygenation as oxygen demands exceed supply. This may result from an increase in metabolic activity by the cell, for example a muscle cell during moderate or strenuous exercise, or by a reduced supply, which is then inadequate to support even basal cell activities.

c Homeostatic restoration of cellular oxygenation as blood supply to the cell is increased. This usually necessitates the dilation of blood vessels, notably arterioles, and the relaxation of precapillary sphincters.

d Failure to meet the oxygen demands of the cells. In exercise this will be transient and is characterized by a 'stitch' and muscle fatigue. As a pathological disorder, for example in intravascular thrombosis, infarction will ensue. Such ischaemic events are associated with pain, presumably because anaerobic metabolism causes the release of pain-producing chemicals from damaged cells.

Shock is characterized by a failure to maintain an adequate supply of oxygen-rich blood to tissues throughout the body, resulting in widespread hypoxia. The cause of this hypoxia is a fall in systemic arterial blood pressure and a reduced cardiac output; that is, a failure to maintain circulatory homeostasis, though it is the inability to maintain metabolic homeostasis within the cells of the body which is ultimately life threatening.

If oxygen supply cannot match cellular requirements, then the generation of ATP declines and that of lactic acid increases. Since ATP is utilized as an energy source in all cells, lack of it will eventually reduce cellular activities. Likewise, the effects of excess lactic acid disrupt protein structure, which will also reduce activities within the cell as enzymes become denatured. This disruption to cells will accelerate as cellular functions deteriorate and, consequently, cell and tissue death will eventually ensue (Figure 5.8). The need for the homeostatic maintenance of tissue oxygenation is therefore clear. In shock, most, if not all, tissues of the body become hypoxic as a consequence of circulatory failure.

As cells lose their structural integrity, a point is reached when the damage is irreversible. If oxygen supply is restored prior to this point, cell function will begin to recover. Beyond this point, however, restoration of tissue oxygenation will produce at most a transient improvement; cell function will then continue to decline. All practitioners should be aware of this progression and the importance of rapid intervention: should a 'shocked' patient enter the irreversible phase then death will result from widespread organ failure.

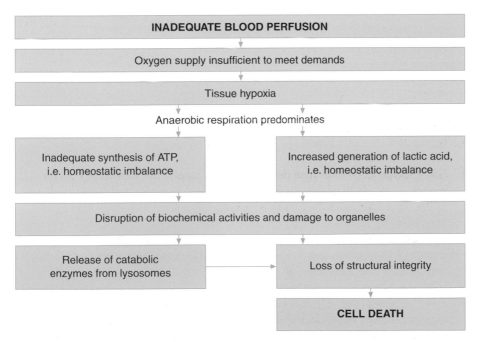

Figure 5.8 **Hypoxia and cell death**

Symptoms of hypoxia

Numerous symptoms are indicative of shock. Those relating directly to the circulatory system are described in the next section (pp. 166–9), but there are others, which arise from hypoxia and the resultant hypoxaemia.

> **EXERCISE**
>
> Using a medical or nursing dictionary, make sure that you are aware of the difference between 'hypoxia' and 'hypoxaemia'.

1   Should the individual remain conscious, there would be neurological symptoms including nausea, dizziness, confusion and anxiety.
2   Hypoxaemia in the vicinity of peripheral chemoreceptors stimulates rapid breathing (i.e. tachypnoea) and this promotes feelings of breathlessness, which further increase anxiety. This will promote increased respiratory effort.
3   As metabolism declines throughout the body, less heat is generated. The transference of heat through the body is also diminished because of the circulatory failure, which occurs in shock. Core temperature therefore declines. In septic shock (see later) body temperature may be initially elevated as severe bacterial infection promotes a pyrexia, but even this is reversed as the shock progresses.
4   There is widespread cyanosis as blood which has pooled in tissues becomes depleted of oxygen. Cyanosis is particularly observable in the nail beds, where it reflects pooling in the extremities.

Hypovolaemic shock

> **EXERCISE**
>
> Before proceeding further, reflect on your understanding of the following terms:
>
> **a** heart rate and stroke volume.
> **b** cardiac output.
> **c** total peripheral resistance.
> **d** blood reservoir.

The most characteristic feature of shock – though this is not always observed in its initial stages – is a profound decrease in arterial (i.e. aortic) blood pressure. Cardiac output and total peripheral resistance determine aortic pressure, a decrease in aortic pressure and its decrease reflects changes in these parameters. There are various types of shock, classified according to the cause of the circulatory disturbance (Figure 5.9). This section considers hypovolaemic shock, which has particular relevance to surgery.

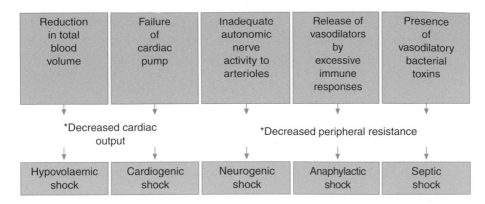

*These are factors in the initial stages. Reductions in both cardiac output and peripheral resistance are eventually features of all types of shock.

Figure 5.9 **Classification of shock by cause of cardiovascular disturbance**

Hypovolaemic shock arises when blood volume is diminished to the point that an adequate cardiac output cannot be maintained. The hypovolaemia may result from loss of whole blood through internal haemorrhage, for example a ruptured spleen, or through external haemorrhage, for example in trauma or surgery, or from the loss of extracellular fluid through burns, vomiting, diarrhoea or excessive diuresis. A decrease in blood volume of 15 to 20 per cent is sufficient to initiate shock.

EXERCISE

How much blood (in an adult) does 20 per cent of the total volume represent, and how does this compare with the volume of a standard blood donation?

Hypovolaemia causes a reduction in cardiac output simply because there is inadequate return of blood to the heart. The effects on aortic pressure are initially minimized because of the effects of increased sympathetic nerve activity, and the actions of various vasoconstrictor hormones, to increase total peripheral resistance. Cardiac responses are also evident, most noticeably an increased heart (pulse) rate, promoted mainly by sympathetic nerve activity. The hypovolaemia means, however, that stroke volume remains reduced, and so the pulse will feel weak ('thready') when palpated (see Box 5.8).

Other responses act to support the circulation during the initial stages of hypovolaemia. Thus, there is a movement of tissue fluid across capillary walls into the blood, which helps to reduce the hypovolaemia. Blood is released by the contraction of blood 'reservoirs', i.e. the spleen and the great veins, redistributing blood so that a greater proportion is now found in the arteries.

All of these compensatory mechanisms have limited capacity. If there is further loss of blood volume then their activities will eventually become inadequate as cardiac output declines yet further. Blood pressure will then begin to fall. Inadequate tissue perfusion causes hypoxia (Figure 5.10) which will be widespread throughout the body. This in turn causes arterioles to dilate, and so reduces peripheral resistance. Blood pressure will then fall rapidly and, without the force to drive it through, blood will pool within the tissues, reducing venous return to the heart, thus exacerbating the circulatory imbalance.

EXERCISE

Hypoxia has localized effects on blood vessels. Using this chapter and the introduction to shock, explain why this action is important in health. (Clue: in health, this process is referred to as 'autoregulation'.)

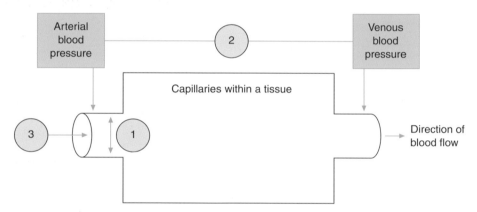

Figure 5.10 **Factors influencing blood perfusion of a tissue**
1   Blood vessel (notably arterioles) diameter. The capacity to alter vessel diameter by dilation or constriction of these vessels provides a means of controlling blood flow.
2   Blood pressure gradient. This provides the force necessary to 'push' blood through the tissue. It is determined primarily by the arterial blood pressure, since venous pressure is normally very small.
3   The availability of adequate blood to perfuse the tissue as required. This is largely determined by the cardiac output but may also involve redistribution of blood from other tissues.

Note
There are other influences on tissue perfusion in ill-health. Thus, factors such as blood viscosity, temperature and vessel length will influence perfusion of the tissues, but these factors are normally constant. The lining of the blood vessels is another factor; roughened surfaces will introduce turbulence and so reduce flow through a vessel. The normal smoothness of the lining reduces the influence of this factor.

Two important points should be noted from this discussion.

1   Cardiac output, blood pressure and tissue perfusion are interdependent. Thus, a decreased cardiac output compromises the homeostatic regulation of systemic arterial blood pressure. A reduced pressure causes a fall in tissue perfusion, leading to hypoxia and, consequently, further vasodilation and the pooling of blood within the tissues. In turn, this causes a reduction in the return of blood to the heart (sometimes referred to as a decreased effective circulating blood volume), so cardiac output will decrease still further. This interdependency is apparent in all forms of shock. What differs is the point of failure, i.e. the maintenance of an adequate cardiac output or the control of peripheral resistance.
2   This relationship between cardiovascular variables means that circulatory disturbance in all types of shock is progressive. The factors that promoted the initial homeostatic disturbance lead to further circulatory decline.

Circulatory symptoms of hypovolaemic shock

Various symptoms arising from tissue hypoxia were noted in a previous section (p. 166). Other symptoms that relate to inadequate blood circulation are also observed, in addition to effects on arterial blood pressure and pulse rate.

1   As shock progresses, the loss of circulation to the skin causes it to become pale and cold. Although cold, the skin may also be clammy because sympathetic nerve activation in response to the hypotension will promote the secretion of sweat.
2   Inadequate renal perfusion will cause urine production to become inadequate and introduce the risk of acute renal failure.
3   Inadequate perfusion of the gastrointestinal tract, together with increased sympathetic nerve activity, will cause a cessation of bowel movement.
4   Inadequate blood circulation, together with a renal disturbance (2, above), will disturb electrolyte distribution in the body, leading to changes in blood composition.
5   Hypoxaemia, and the presence of damaged cells within the tissues, will promote blood clotting, thus disseminated intravascular coagulation (DIC) is a risk in shock.

EXERCISE

Blood clotting is a complex process and has to be triggered.
Review the relevant sections in the previous chapter and answer the following questions.

1   How do damaged cells promote the clotting process?
2   What is the positive feedback that aids haemostasis?

Box 5.12   Application: the prevention of shock

Pre-operative assessment

The pre-operative assessment and preparation of any patient is an essential part of any surgical procedure. Where possible, surgery should be carried out under optimal conditions, in order to reduce the risk of problems occurring during the perioperative phase. In emergency situations, this may not always be possible.

During the pre-operative assessment fitness for anaesthesia and surgery are assessed, particular attention is paid to the cardiovascular system, respiratory system and renal disorders. Any drug therapy such as anticoagulants, steroids, insulin and drugs used to treat cardiac failure or hypertension is also of particular importance. Allergic and hypersensitive reactions to drugs and other agents must be noted.

A physical assessment is carried out on the cardiovascular system, the respiratory system and general metabolic status, including a haematological and biochemical assessment. If the patient requires any treatment to ensure optimum fitness pre-operatively, such as blood transfusion or chest physiotherapy, this must be achieved prior to admission.

In emergency situations it may still be possible to perform a pre-operative assessment. If the patient is hypovolaemic then blood volume must be restored before anaesthesia commences, the exception being when there is life threatening haemorrhage, or another contraindication.

The perioperative phase

Hypovolaemic shock is the most common form of shock during the perioperative phase: close monitoring of the blood pressure, cardiac output, blood loss, urine and gastrointestinal fluid loss are essential in the early detection of hypovolaemia.

Some monitoring may already be in place before the patient reaches the anaesthetic room, for example in emergency situations; otherwise it is common practice for the monitoring equipment to be attached to the patient in the anaesthetic room. Early monitoring provides valuable information on the patient's haemodynamic condition and cardiac function.

It is important to have good venous access for drug and fluid administration.

Oxygen therapy to provide adequate tissue perfusion is essential. Pulse oximetry provides an indication of the oxygen saturation of the haemoglobin; however, it is slow to respond to hypoxia and cyanosis might be seen before the pulse oximetry changes.

Blood pressure

Measurement is achieved by using either an indirect automatic blood pressure monitor, which can make measurements at frequent intervals, or by measuring the arterial pressure directly by inserting a cannula into a suitable artery and monitoring the pressure via tubing to a pressure display unit. A fall in blood pressure is an indication of shock, when it is combined with a weakening rapid pulse.

Electrocardiogram monitoring is used to detect arrhythmias (see Figure 5.4) and myocardial ischaemia. Central venous catheterization provides an accurate measurement of the central venous pressure (see Box 5.9), and allows for the safe administration of intravenous fluids avoiding inadvertent over-transfusion (see Chapter 3).

Core temperature monitoring provides information upon thermoregulation, skin temperature reflects peripheral perfusion and the difference between the central and peripheral temperature indicates the degree of vasoconstriction and vasodilation.

Fluid administration

The initial type of fluid replacement therapy in the treatment of shock is often a 'colloid' and/or 'crystalloid' fluid. At a later stage, usually following blood cross-matching, red blood cells may be needed. In routine surgical cases, the patient's blood will have been cross-matched at the pre-operative assessment stage and, where blood loss during surgery could be high, e.g. in bowel or vascular surgery, donor blood will be cross-matched and be available for use. For a full description of the principals of infusate therapy, see Chapter 3. Dilution of clotting factors can occur following the infusion of large amounts of fluids. This may need to be corrected by transfusion of fresh frozen plasma, and/or platelets.

Insertion of a urinary catheter ensures accurate urine measurement; the catheter should be connected to a graduated collecting device. Urine output can be measured at regular intervals giving an indication of renal function.

Metabolic assessment and regulation

In the case of routine surgery all patients should have been assessed pre-operatively and their general metabolic status established; in emergency surgery this needs to be established as soon as possible. However, during all types of surgical procedures it may become necessary to review the situation at regular intervals. Initial glucose, urea and electrolyte levels are required to establish a baseline, and arterial pH and blood gas measurements are required to assess for signs of hypoxia, hypercapnia and acid base balance. Lactate levels provide a good indication of cellular hypoxia and hepatic function.

It is very important that effective analgesia is achieved. Morphine is the treatment of choice, and is given intravenously in increments every two to five minutes until pain is controlled. This ensures safe administration, which should not alter the conscious level of the patient, but will help to reduce anxiety (Carrie *et al.* 1997).

The role of the theatre team

Accurate measurement of all fluid loss and administration is essential. The anaesthetist will carefully monitor all fluids administered; any changes in the vital signs will determine the rate and type of fluids given to the patient. The theatre practitioner is trained to anticipate untoward events, like a decline in patient condition, responding promptly and efficiently.

The surgical team use careful surgical techniques like surgical diathermy, bowel bags, moist 45 cm by 45 cm swabs, in order to minimize blood and fluid loss during surgery.

In emergency situations the surgical team will work quickly to prevent further fluid loss. The 'scrub' person has to be aware of all fluid loss and keep a careful note of the amount of irrigation fluids as they are used. All fluid output is measured; this includes the blood loss on swabs, the contents of suction bottles, urine measurement, faecal fluid and gastric contents. A running total of all fluid loss must be maintained to ensure accurate fluid replacement therapy.

Epidural and spinal analgesia

Epidural and spinal analgesia impairs the sympathetic outflow from the spinal cord and can cause a profound fall in the blood pressure (see Chapter 8, pp. 254–60). When hypovolaemia is present, peripheral vasoconstriction occurs in an attempt to maintain blood pressure.

Post-operative phase

Post-operative management will depend on the physical condition of the patient. If the patient has experienced uncomplicated hypovolaemic shock and is in a stable condition, the patient will be managed in the recovery ward. Fluid replacement therapy, monitoring of vital signs and pain management will be continued. Patients who have suffered severe trauma, sepsis and cardiogenic shock or have other secondary complications, may require intensive care immediately post-operatively, with the provision of advanced cardiovascular, respiratory and renal support. The main principles of intervention in the correction of hypovolaemic shock are shown in Table 5.2.

Table 5.2 Restoration of homeostasis by clinical intervention in hypovolaemic shock

Homeostatic disturbance	Correction of disturbance	Monitoring
Hypoxaemia	• Supplemental O_2 (with intubation if necessary)	• Evaluation of airway • Observation of respiratory pattern for signs of change • Chest radiography for signs of secretions
Hypotension/ low cardiac output	• Replacement of lost fluid by blood, red cells, plasma expanders, or electrolyte infusions, or as required • Elevate extremities to increase venous return • Inotropic drugs to increase myocardial contractility • Pneumatic anti-shock garment to increase peripheral resistance	• Regular (5–15 minute) observation of arterial blood pressure, skin colour and temperature • Monitoring of central venous pressure • Monitor in-dwelling catheters • Trend analysis
Blood electrolyte disturbance	• Replacement by mixed electrolyte infusion	• Laboratory values
Neurological disturbance	• Reassurance to reduce anxiety • Symptoms should reduce with control of other symptoms	• Level of consciousness
Oliguria	• Should improve with circulatory improvement	• Intake vs. output trends (output at least 1 ml of urine/kg body wt/hour) • Urinalysis • In-dwelling catheter cares
Hypothermia	• Hyperthemic blanket • Warming lights • Use of warmed infusates	• Warming must be gradual • Monitor core and skin temperature every 30–60 minutes
Clotting disturbance	• Blood replacement will restore clotting factors	• Coagulation profile of blood samples • Observe for signs of disseminated intravascular coagulation
Bowel stasis	• Should improve with circulatory improvement	• No oral food to be taken until bowel sounds are heard

Summary

- The cardiovascular system is the body's transport network.
- The heart provides the pumping action necessary to support the circulation, by ensuring that there is adequate blood to perfuse the tissues, and also by generating the pressure necessary to drive the circulation. Cardiac function is modified by the autonomic nervous system and the endocrine system, and such extrinsic influences are largely responsible for the control of cardiac output at rest and when the circulation is challenged during, for example, exercise or haemorrhage.
- Arteries are the distributing vessels of the circulatory system, capillaries enable nutrient and 'waste' exchange with tissue cells to ensure intracellular homeostasis occurs, and veins are drainage vessels and blood reservoirs.
- Blood flow through a tissue is determined by the blood pressure differential between arterial and venous vessels and by the peripheral resistance provided by the vasculature, particularly arterioles.
- Arterial blood pressure provides the force necessary to produce blood flow, and is itself determined by the cardiac output and the total peripheral resistance. The pressure is normally maintained within its homeostatic range via a number of short-term and long-term blood pressure homeostatic controls. Sympathetic nerve activity is of particular importance as a short-term regulator, whilst various hormones support its actions, and also influence blood volume.
- Drugs used when cardiovascular function is compromised are classed as chronotrophic and inotropic drugs (i.e. affect the heart rate and strength of contractility respectively), and vasodilator and vasoconstrictor drugs which have an effect on blood vessel diameter and hence blood pressure.
- Shock is a serious condition arising through a failure to maintain cardiovascular function, and hence a failure to maintain tissue oxygen homeostasis. It is a clinical emergency and, if not reversed quickly enough, is progressive and fatal.
- There are five main types of shock, classified according to the cause of the initial cardiovascular imbalance. However, there is commonality of symptoms as the circulatory failure progresses. Interventions are directed at supporting the circulation and blood oxygenation until the underlying cause of the problem can be corrected.
- Regular, accurate monitoring is vital; the risk of shock occurring during surgery can be reduced by good nursing practice, including keen observation of the patient. Monitoring techniques have a particularly valuable role to play; the astute observation of the condition of the patient is an effective means of avoiding this major disturbance of systemic and cellular homeostasis.

Bibliography

Autar, R. (1999) Huntleigh Healthcare clinical feature supplement: deep vein thrombosis: a risky business. *British Journal of Perioperative Nursing* 9(3): 114–15.

Bucher, H.C., Hengstler, P., Schindler, C. and Guyatt, G.H. (2000) Percutaneous transluminal coronary angioplasty versus medical treatment for non-acute coronary heart disease: meta-analysis of randomized controlled trials. *BMJ* 321(7253): 73–7.

Burton, J. (2000) Oscillometric blood pressure monitors. *British Journal of Perioperative Nursing* 10(12): 624–6.

Carrie, L.E.S., Simpson, P.J. and Popat, M.T. (1997) *Understanding Anaesthesia, Third Edition*. Oxford: Butterworth Heinemann.

Clancy, J. and McVicar, A.J. (2002) *Physiology and Anatomy. A Homeostatic Approach, Second Edition*. London: Arnold.

Colletti, C. (1999) Emergency! Pericarditis. *American Journal of Nursing* 99(10): 35.

Criley, J.M. (1999) Bits & bytes of PA education. The physiological origins of heart sounds and murmurs: the unique interactive guide to cardiac diagnosis. *Perspective on Physician Assistant Education* 10(3): 152.

Cucherat, M., Bonnefoy, E. and Tremeau, G. (2001) Primary angioplasty versus intravenous thrombolysis for acute myocardial infarction. Oxford: The Cochran Library. Issue 1.

Darovic, G.A. and Franklin, C.M. (1999) *Handbook of Hemodynamic Monitoring*. London: W.B. Saunders.
This interdisciplinary handbook covers both the fundamentals and advanced concepts of invasive and non-invasive hemodynamic monitoring technologies and their practical applications to clinical practice in a portable format.

Goh, T.H. (2000) Common congenital heart defects: the value of early detection. *Australian Family Physician* 29(5): 429–31, 434–5, 462–3.

Griffiths, R. (2000) Back to basics: anaesthesia: circulation and invasive monitoring. *British Journal of Perioperative Nursing* 10(3): 167–71.

Heuther, S.E. and McCance, K.L. (1996) *Understanding Pathophysiology*. London: Mosby.

Hood, W.B. Jr., Dans, A., Guyatt, G.H., Jaeschke, R. and McMurray, J. (2001) Digitalis for treatment of congestive heart failure in patients in sinus rhythm. Oxford: The Cochran Library. Issue 1.

Lilly, T.K. and Rupp, T. (2001) Sac attack: pathophysiology, assessment & prehospital treatment of cardiac tamponade. *JEMS: Journal of Emergency Medical Services* 26(4): 58–60, 62–4, 66–75.

Lipton, B. (2000) Estimation of central venous pressure by ultrasound of the internal jugular vein. *American Journal of Emergency Medicine* 18(4): 432–4.

MacKlin, M. (2001) Managing heart failure: a case study approach. *Critical Care Nurse* 21(2): 36–8, 40–6, 48 passim.

Miracle, V.A. (2001) Put the brakes on pericarditis: learn what to do when the sac surrounding your patient's heart is inflamed. *Nursing* 31(4): 44–5.

Morrill, P. (2000) Pharmacotherapeutics of positive inotropes. *AORN Journal* 71(1): 173–8, 181–8, 190–2.

Nagle, B.M. and O'Keefe, L.M. (1999) Closing in on mitral valve disease. *Nursing* 29(4): 32–7.

Neal, M.J. (1997) *Medical Pharmacology at a Glance, Third Edition*. Oxford: Blackwell Science.

Oeltjen, A.M. and Santrach, P.J. (1997) Autologous transfusion techniques. *Journal of Intravenous Nursing* 20(6): 305–10.

Pradka, L.R. (2000) Lipids and their role in coronary heart disease: what they do and how to manage them. *Nursing Clinics of North America* 35(4): 981–91.

Rankin, S. (1996) Managing hypovolaemic shock. *British Journal of Theatre Nursing* 6(2): 10–1.

Richardson, D.A., Bexton, R., Shaw, F.E., Steen, N., Bond, J. and Kenny, R.A. (2000) Complications of carotid sinus massage – a prospective series of older patients. *Age & Ageing* 29(5): 413–17.

Seal, J. (2000) Clinical feature article: autologous blood transfusions. *British Journal of Perioperative Nursing* 10(4): 194–8.

Spence, M. (2000) Clinical feature article: beating heart coronary artery bypass grafting: a theatre nurse's perspective. *British Journal of Perioperative Nursing* 10(3): 138–43.

Warsaw, D.S., Niewiarowska, A. and Theman, T. (2000) Effect of autotransfusion on fibrinolysis in open heart patients. *Journal of Extra-Corporeal Technology* 32(1): 20–4.

Williams, M.J., Clancy, J. and McVicar, A.J. (eds) (2001) Know your heart. *British Journal of Perioperative Nursing*.

Answers to multiple choice questions

Q.2, p. 160

a Spurts from the proximal side of the wound.

Q.2, p. 160

b The pulse rate increases and the blood pressure falls.

Chapter 6

Perioperative influences on respiratory homeostasis

Introduction

'Respiration' and 'breathing' are terms that tend to be used interchangeably in relation to the role of the respiratory system. Strictly speaking, the term 'respiration' is most appropriately applied to those biochemical reactions that are involved in energy production within cells, entailing the breakdown of glucose using oxygen, and producing carbon dioxide and water in the process. Oxygen is obtained from the air we breathe, and carbon dioxide is excreted into it and so the functioning of the lungs clearly also has a role in respiratory processes. Distinction is sometimes made between these two aspects by referring to the cellular reactions as 'internal' respiration and lung functioning as 'external' respiration. 'Breathing', of course, relates to the latter.

The chemical reactions that comprise 'internal' respiration may be summarized as follows:

$$6O_2 + C_6H_{12}O_6 \longrightarrow 6CO_2 + 6H_2O \ (+ \ Energy) \quad (6.1)$$
$$\text{oxygen} \quad \text{glucose} \qquad\qquad \text{carbon} \quad \text{water}$$
$$\text{dioxide}$$

Whilst production of carbon dioxide is normal, excess gas must be excreted to prevent an accumulation of harmful carbonic acid arising from the reaction of the gas with water:

$$CO_2 + H_2O \ \underset{\longleftarrow}{\longrightarrow} \ H_2CO_3 \ \underset{\longleftarrow}{\longrightarrow} \ H^+ + HCO_3^- \quad (6.2)$$
$$\text{carbon} \quad \text{water} \qquad \text{carbonic} \qquad \text{hydrogen} \quad \text{bicarbonate}$$
$$\text{dioxide} \qquad\qquad \text{acid} \qquad\qquad \text{ions} \qquad \text{ions}$$

As time elapses high levels of carbon dioxide in the blood would also cause an increase in heart rate and irritability of the heart muscle. There might also be an increase in the blood pressure and blood flow to the brain, eventually leading to coma and respiratory depression.

EXERCISE

Find out how much oxygen is utilized each minute by the body at rest.

- If oxygen comprises 21 per cent of the air we breathe, how much air should we breathe to support this utilization rate?
- Define the terms 'dyspnoea' and 'apnoea'.

Disturbances of blood gas homeostasis are frequent complications in both the surgical and medical fields. The usual problems are outlined below.

- A deficiency of oxygen in the tissues, referred to as 'hypoxia' (hypo- = less than normal). In the absence of anaemia or circulatory disorder, hypoxia will usually have its origin in the lungs. Thus, the oxygenation of blood is compromised, producing 'hypoxaemia' (-aemia = of the blood). The terms 'hypoxia' and 'hypoxaemia' are often used interchangeably. Although this is not strictly correct, hypoxaemia does promote tissue hypoxia and so 'hypoxia' tends to be the preferred term. Hypoxia prevents cells from performing normal aerobic respiration (aer- = using air), causing an increased reliance on anaerobic (anaer- = without air) respiration which is less efficient and potentially harmful.
- Excessive carbon dioxide in the tissues, referred to as 'hypercapnia' (hyper- = more than normal). Hypercapnia may also arise from circulatory or lung problems, but may also reflect excessive carbon dioxide production by metabolically-active tissues. Hypercapnia is problematic because it causes increased generation of carbonic acid (see Equation 6.2, above), leading to excessive acidity. The involvement of carbon dioxide would make this a respiratory acidosis (Box 6.1), as distinct from the metabolic acidosis arising from other (metabolic) sources.

As noted earlier, it is the respiratory system, comprised of the lungs and associated structures (Figure 6.1), that provides the means of taking up oxygen from the environment, and excreting carbon dioxide into it. Our lungs basically are organs that provide a large surface area, and as thin a barrier as possible, for adequate gas exchange to occur between blood and air. The airways within the lungs terminate in minute clusters of cup-shaped or globular sacs called alveoli (approximately 300 million in total), that provide a surface area equivalent to approximately two football pitches. Alveoli are richly supplied with blood capillaries and the barrier formed by the capillary endothelial membrane and the alveolar epithelial membrane forms the barrier across which gases must exchange between the lung and blood.

The blood conveys oxygen to the tissues, from which it picks up carbon dioxide and returns this to the lungs. The carriage of the gases by blood is therefore central to respiratory functioning. It is the processes involved in blood gas homeostasis, and the impact that surgery may have on those processes, that form the focus of this chapter.

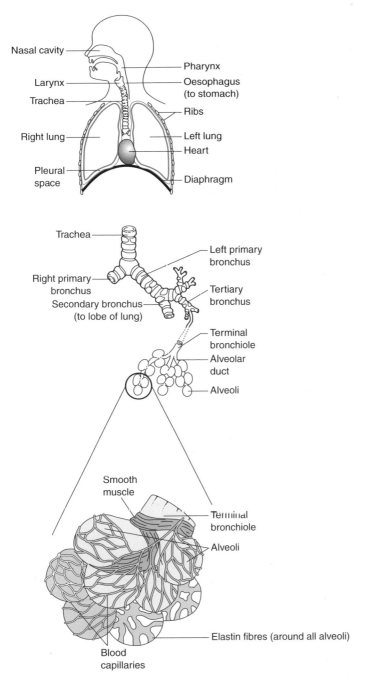

Figure 6.1 **The respiratory 'tree'**

Q. What happens to the amount of cartilage present on passing from the top of the trachea to the alveoli?

> **Box 6.1   Application: respiratory acidosis and alkalosis**
>
> These terms were defined and explained in Chapter 3 (Box 3.5). Respiratory dysfunction typically produces 'respiratory' acidosis, or alkalosis, because the disturbance arises from too much or too little carbon dioxide, respectively, in the body fluids. This gas generates carbonic acid, and hence hydrogen ions.
>
> Given time, the body may produce a degree of compensation by altering the urinary excretion of hydrogen ions and bicarbonate ions (which act to 'buffer' hydrogen ions – see Chapter 3), and in this way help to provide partial restoration of body fluid pH. However, the compensation requires a few days to be effective and so is unlikely to be observed perioperatively, where disturbances are likely to be acute.
>
> Acid–base disturbances also have other non-respiratory causes. For example, excessive diarrhoea may result in the loss of so many bicarbonate ions (i.e. base) that an acidosis occurs. Conversely, the loss of excessive amounts of gastric acid may induce an alkalosis. Such disturbances are referred to as 'metabolic' changes to acid–base balance. Diarrhoea and vomiting in the perioperative period were considered in detail in Chapter 3.

EXERCISE

It is not within the scope of this chapter to describe the structure of the respiratory system in detail, but it is necessary that the reader is familiar with the general anatomy of the airways. Figure 6.1 is provided for reference.

What do you think might be the roles of the pleural membranes and the fluid-filled pleural space?

To answer this you might consider the potential for lung damage from frictional rub during breathing, but also the need to maintain adhesion of the lungs to the chest wall.

Principles of blood gas homeostasis

Partial pressures of gases

Oxygen and carbon dioxide are both carried by blood in gaseous form and in combination with other chemicals. In particular, the carriage of gases is facilitated by their combination with the pigment haemoglobin, present in red blood cells. Haemoglobin consists of a protein called globin, and a pigment called haem. Haem molecules can reversibly bind with oxygen, whilst the globin part of the haemoglobin molecule can reversibly combine with carbon dioxide or hydrogen ions; globin therefore has an important role in the transportation of carbon dioxide by blood, and in the regulation of blood acidity.

The carriage of gases by blood is complex. One common factor, however, is that the total amounts of either oxygen and carbon dioxide that may be carried in a given volume of normal blood is determined by the pressure that is exerted by that gas which is in gaseous form and simply dissolved in the plasma/blood cells.

We can easily observe that dissolved gases exert a pressure by opening a bottle of fizzy drink. The dissolved carbon dioxide quickly forms bubbles as the pressure is released and the gas escapes. But what of a mixture of gases? According to Dalton's Law, individual constituent gases each contributes to the total pressure of the mixed gas according to their individual proportions. The pressure exerted by an individual gas within a mixture is referred to as its 'partial pressure'. This concept is explored in more detail later when gas exchange between lung and blood is discussed. For now it is sufficient to note that the partial pressure of oxygen dissolved in blood leaving the lungs averages 13.3 kiloPascals (kPa[1]), whilst that of carbon dioxide averages 5.3 kPa.

Carriage of oxygen by blood

Oxygen is poorly soluble in blood plasma, and so haemoglobin is vital for its transport. In fact, almost 99 per cent of the oxygen found in oxygenated blood is transported in combination with haemoglobin (oxyhaemoglobin), and the dissolved gas accounts for only 1 per cent of the total amount of oxygen present. Functionally, haemoglobin must bind reversibly with oxygen, otherwise the gas will not be released in the tissues. The local partial pressure of oxygen is the determining factor. In the lungs, the partial pressure of oxygen is relatively high and haemoglobin rapidly picks up the gas. As a consequence, blood leaves the lungs with its haemoglobin virtually saturated (over 97 per cent). Indeed the affinity is such that blood would still be almost saturated with oxygen if the partial pressure of oxygen is even less than the average 13.3 kPa. This accounts for the 'plateau' phase of the oxygen–haemoglobin dissociation curve (Figure 6.2).

The partial pressure of oxygen in blood within the tissues is reduced as the gas is utilized (Figure 6.2). The lower pressure represents less dissolved gas and this causes it to dissociate from the oxyhaemoglobin. In this way more of the gas becomes available to the tissue cells. Conditions associated with high metabolic activity, i.e. increased tissue temperature and acidity, act to further improve the release of oxygen from haemoglobin and so helps to facilitate the elevated metabolic rate of the tissue concerned. This adaptation to metabolism is referred to as the 'Bohr effect', after the physiologist Christian Bohr (1855–1911) who first noted it.

[1] The fundamental unit of pressure is called a Pascal (1000 Pascals = 1 kiloPascal). Use of this unit is now standard for gas pressures. Arterial blood pressure continues to be measured in millimetres of mercury (or centimetres of water for venous pressure), which is a derived unit of pressure based simply on what fluid is present in the sphygmomanometer. Suggestions have already been made in science circles that blood pressure measurements should also be recorded in Pascals.

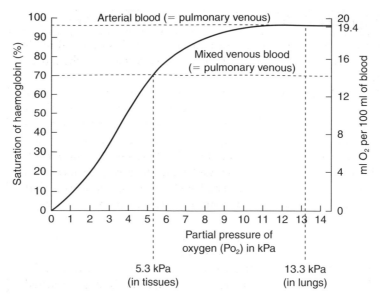

Figure 6.2 **The oxygen–haemoglobin dissociation curve**
See text, p. 181, for explanation

Q. What is the saturation of haemoglobin when the partial pressure of oxygen is 4.5 kPa?

Carriage of carbon dioxide by blood

The usage of oxygen within tissues yields carbon dioxide (see Equation 6.1). Similarly to oxygen, only a relatively small amount of carbon dioxide is carried simply as dissolved gas, though carbon dioxide is the more soluble of the two gases and so the actual proportion is much higher for carbon dioxide than it is for oxygen (7 per cent and 1 per cent respectively). Again the partial pressure produced by the dissolved gas (about 6.0 kPa; this is higher than that in arterial blood because the blood has gained carbon dioxide) encourages the combination of carbon dioxide with other chemicals, including haemoglobin. In contrast to the carriage of oxygen, only about 23 per cent of the carbon dioxide will be carried by haemoglobin (in a form referred to as carbamino-haemoglobin). Most (70 per cent) carbon dioxide carried by blood is found combined with water to form bicarbonate ions (see Equation 6.2). This reaction between the gas and water makes carbon dioxide even more soluble in water than the dissolved gas proportion might suggest.

When blood reaches the lungs, the carbon dioxide must be released from its various forms and once again the local partial pressure is the determining factor; it is lower in lung alveoli than in blood returning to the lung and so the dissolved carbon dioxide diffuses out of the blood. As the dissolved component diminishes, other sources give up their carbon dioxide and some of this will also then diffuse

Box 6.2 Application: pulse oximetry

Accurate measurement of the oxygen saturation of blood is essential in all perioperative circumstances. This can be reliably achieved with the aid of pulse oximetry.

Blood entering the capillaries of skin normally yields only a little of its oxygen because skin is not a very active tissue. Consequently, blood passing through the tissue will have almost the same composition as arterial blood entering it, since the degree of oxygen extraction becomes very small in comparison with the amount of blood present. The saturation of blood with oxygen (abbreviated as SaO_2) therefore can be measured from a finger using a pulse oximeter. The benefit of pulse oximetry is that it is non-invasive and it provides a continual assessment of blood oxygenation.

Patients should be attached to a pulse oximeter during all stages of the perioperative period; this includes patients who are undergoing procedures with conscious sedation. The effectiveness of oxygen therapy can be assessed and appropriate action taken if hypoxaemia is not corrected (O'Reilly 2000).

If ventilation of the lungs, and the uptake of oxygen from them, is sufficiently poor to reduce the oxygen saturation then this could be expected to change the pulse oximetry reading, and so the method might be used to monitor lung function. However, factors such as anaemia and the efficiency of the peripheral circulation must also be taken into account. For example, a localized reduction of blood flow to the finger to which the oximeter is attached will cause the reading to decrease, irrespective of how well the lungs are functioning. In addition, pulse oximeters are slow to respond and so should be supported by use of good observational assessment (e.g. looking for signs of developing cyanosis).

Pulse oximetry is considered to be one of the most significant clinical aids to care that have been introduced in recent years. A useful text for those readers who wish to explore the use of pulse oximetry in more detail is that by Moyle, Hahn and Adams (1998).

EXERCISE

Using pulse oximetry, a saturation of 90 per cent plus is considered adequate. Refer to Figure 6.2 and explain why this is so.

into the alveoli. This includes the conversion of bicarbonate ions back to carbon dioxide, a process facilitated by an enzyme called carbonic anhydrase.

It is important to note the relatively high solubility of carbon dioxide compared to that of oxygen. This is because a slight change in the partial pressure of the gas in blood reflects a significantly greater change in the amount of carbon dioxide that is present. For example, Figure 6.2 illustrates that a decrease in the partial pressure of oxygen in arterial blood from the 'normal' 13.3 kPa to about 10.5 kPa has only a small effect on the volume of oxygen carried because it remains near-saturated. In contrast, a similar proportionate increase in the partial pressure of carbon dioxide, from 5.3 kPa to 6.4 kPa, would represent an almost 20 per cent increase in the carbon dioxide content, and lead to a significant increase in body fluid acidity (via carbonic acid; see Equation 6.2).

Lung function and blood gas homeostasis

The discussion so far has identified two crucial aspects of blood gas homeostasis. First, since oxygen and carbon dioxide in blood are carried mainly in combination with other constituents of blood, these combinations must be reversible to enable loading and unloading as appropriate. Second, the factor that determines the combination or release of the gases is the partial pressure exerted by the gas simply dissolved in the blood.

It is this second point that illustrates the importance of the lungs, since it is the gas exchange here that determines the partial pressures of the gases within blood. In fact, the partial pressure of oxygen and carbon dioxide in blood leaving the lungs matches that of the gases within the lungs themselves. This is a key point since it explains why lung functioning must be rigorously controlled. Failure to maintain that control, or to permit normal gas exchange across the lung–blood barrier, will induce alterations to the partial pressures of gases within blood and hence in the amount of gas carried by blood.

Alveolar ventilation and the control of breathing

The discussion so far has considered lung function only from the perspective of breathing patterns in relation to maintaining blood gas homeostasis. In fact, the total volume of air that enters the lungs each minute (referred to as the 'pulmonary ventilation rate', or 'pulmonary minute volume') does not equate with the ventilation rate of the alveoli, where gas exchange takes place. This is because not all of the air breathed in passes to the alveoli. Thus, in an adult at rest, only about 350 ml of each breath volume of 500 ml of air reaches the alveoli; the rest remains within the major airways, that is in the pharynx, trachea, bronchi and bronchioles. As these latter areas do not take part in gas exchange they comprise an anatomical 'dead space'. This is an important consideration in clinical situations such as anaesthesia (Box 6.3).

Apart from an effect on the proportion of air breathed that gains access to alveoli, the presence of the dead space also means that the air will mix with gas that has remained in the dead space areas following the previous breath, together with that remaining in the alveoli. Collectively, the anatomical dead space and the gas left in alveoli after a normal expiration at rest comprises a reference value called the 'functional residual capacity' or FRC (Figure 6.3). In an adult, this would be approximately 2 litres. A normal breath at rest is called a 'tidal volume' and in adults averages about 0.5 litres (7–8 ml per kg body weight) and, hence, is relatively small in comparison to the FRC. As a consequence, the composition of

---

Box 6.3   Application: dead space and inhalational anaesthesia

The dead space is increased by the use of masks, and by tubing for assisted ventilation and induction of anaesthesia using inhalational drugs. This increased volume must be taken into account when determining the volume of delivery, and the composition of inspired air (gas), otherwise the required change in alveolar gas composition will not be achieved.

---

alveolar gas after inhalation is very different to that of the air that is inhaled. To consider this further, it is necessary to first clarify the partial pressures of gases in air and in the alveoli, since the two are not of the same composition.

Standard atmospheric pressure is 101 kPa and, since 21 per cent of dry air is comprised of oxygen, the partial pressure of oxygen (PO_2) will be:

$$PO_2 = 21 \times 101/100 = 21 \, kPa \, approx.$$

Only 0.03 per cent of dry air is carbon dioxide, and so its partial pressure will be:

$$PCO_2 = 0.03 \times 101/100 = 0.03 \, kPa \, approx.$$

Most of the remaining pressure is due to nitrogen (dry air is approximately 79 per cent nitrogen). This gas is inert and not normally considered in relation to physiological function.

EXERCISE

If the proportion of air that is nitrogen is 79 per cent, what will be its partial pressure (assuming a standard atmospheric pressure)?

a 89 kPa.
b 79 kPa.
c 69 kPa.
d 59 kPa.

The gas within the lung alveoli will also be at atmospheric pressure after inhalation. Upon inhalation, however, the air will mix with FRC gas that is deficient in oxygen and enriched with carbon dioxide, and will also pick up water vapour from within the moistened airways. The partial pressure of water vapour must be taken into account, together with the altered proportions of oxygen and carbon dioxide. As a result, the partial pressure of oxygen within the alveoli is less than it is in room air: on inhalation it increases to an average of only 13.3 kPa, whilst the partial pressure of carbon dioxide decreases but remains much higher than it is in room air, about 5.3 kPa. These values will change if breathing rate and/or depth are altered since such an altered breathing pattern would influence the alveolar ventilation, and hence gas composition. Breathing movements must therefore be controlled, appropriate to maintain the homeostatic ranges for oxygen and carbon dioxide.

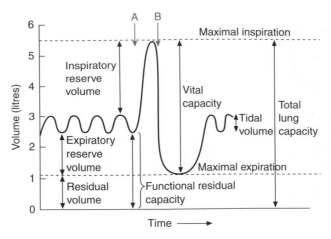

Figure 6.3 **A spirogram to show lung volumes and capacities**
A trace will be obtained by an individual breathing into a spirometer, including taking a deep breath at A and forcibly breathing out at B. Clearly not of wide usage for patient assessment – the diagram is illustrative only. Note the Functional Residual Capacity; see text, pp. 184–5, for explanation and relevance

Q. From this diagram, approximately what are the volumes of the vital capacity, and the Functional Residual Capacity?

Box 6.4   Application: P_aO_2 or P_AO_2?

Abbreviated terms can confuse, including those used in relation to blood gases. This section has recognized the partial pressure of gases within alveoli as well as in blood. Blood gas analysis identifies those values for oxygen and carbon dioxide in blood samples and records them as P_aO_2 and P_aCO_2, respectively. The small 'a' denotes *a*rterial blood. If alveolar gas analysis is performed, the abbreviations P_AO_2 and P_ACO_2 are used, in which the capital 'A' is used to denote *a*lveoli.

Note: If reference is made to the terms S_aO_2 and S_vO_2 then these refer to the 'saturation' of oxygen (expressed as a percentage) in arterial or mixed venous blood, respectively. Venous gas composition is rarely performed; the values are not helpful normally since it is the systemic arterial blood that supplies the tissues of the body.

Breathing movements are largely involuntary and are produced by the rhythmical discharge of nerve impulses from the respiratory centres of the brain stem (Figure 6.4). The impulses pass down the spinal cord to the diaphragm (via the phrenic nerves) and to the intercostal muscles (via intercostal nerves); accessory muscles may also be involved during exertion. The breathing process would be self-defeating if the respiratory muscles themselves were to utilize much of the oxygen taken in during inspiration simply to sustain the movements required to inflate or

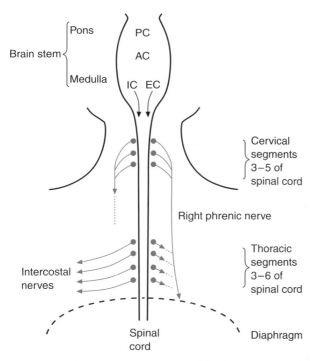

Figure 6.4 **The respiratory centres of the brain stem and nerve supply to the respiratory muscles**
PC = Pneumotaxic centre
AC = Apneustic centre
IC = Inspiratory centre
EC = Expiratory centre
Impulses to the muscles of breathing originate from the IC and EC, but the final neural output is controlled by the PC and AC.

Q. Why are these referred to as 'efferent' or 'motor' nerves?

'deflate' the lungs. In fact, the energy requirements of the lung are very small. During a normal resting inspiration/expiration cycle diaphragmatic movement is sufficient to support inspiration, and expiration is entirely passive through elastic recoil of the lungs and diaphragm. The minimal muscle contraction required at rest means that the lungs consume less than 1 per cent of the total uptake of oxygen. The low energy requirements are facilitated by very low airway resistance (i.e. air flows through them easily) and by the high elasticity of the lungs (i.e. they have a high compliance).

The basic control (i.e. in the absence of exercise, voluntary change, sighing, yawning and coughing) of the rate and depth of breathing relates to the information passing to the respiratory centres of the brain stem from chemoreceptors (i.e. chemically-sensitive receptors; see Figure 6.5) that respond to the local gas composition. The mechanism conforms to the general plan of an intrinsic, homeostatic process that was identified in Chapter 1:

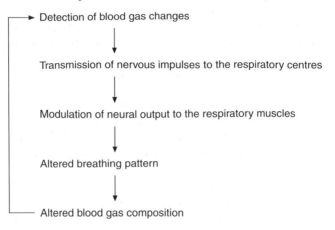

Detection of blood gas changes

↓

Transmission of nervous impulses to the respiratory centres

↓

Modulation of neural output to the respiratory muscles

↓

Altered breathing pattern

↓

Altered blood gas composition

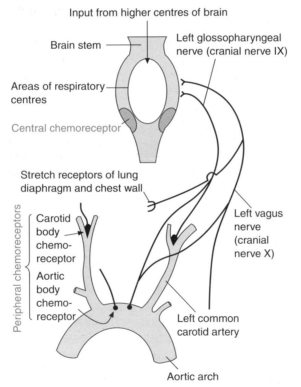

Figure 6.5 **The chemoreceptors and sensory input into the respiratory centres of the brain stem**

Q. What are the advantages of having receptors monitoring arterial, rather than venous, gas composition?

The previous section highlighted that changes in the pressure of carbon dioxide in blood are likely to have a greater consequence for the body than changes in the pressure of oxygen (unless these are especially pronounced). Consequently, it is not surprising to find that the chemoreceptors are more sensitive to the local carbon dioxide composition, and that it is carbon dioxide that provides the main stimulus to alter lung function, and hence alveolar ventilation.

The chemoreceptors are located centrally and peripherally.

1   *Central chemoreceptors*. These receptors are found in the medulla oblongata of the brain stem, close to the respiratory centres (Figure 6.5). They do not actually monitor blood gases directly, but monitor the acidity of the cerebrospinal fluid, or CSF. The CSF is separated from the circulatory system by the 'blood–brain barrier'. This secretory epithelium is impervious to hydrogen ions in the blood but is freely permeable to carbon dioxide and so an increase in the partial pressure of carbon dioxide in arterial blood will cause the gas to diffuse into the CSF, form carbonic acid, and so activate the chemoreceptors. As they are located outside the circulatory system, their responses are relatively slow. They appear to be involved in determining the main, underlying respiratory rhythm.

2   *Peripheral chemoreceptors*. These chemoreceptors are found within the walls of the aortic arch and at the bifurcation of each of the common carotid arteries in the neck (areas called the carotid bodies; see Figure 6.5). An increase in the partial pressure of carbon dioxide (and hence acidity) of arterial blood will stimulate these receptors, and impulses are relayed to the brain stem. These receptors respond rapidly to changes in the partial pressure of carbon dioxide in arterial blood and seem to be involved in rapid, moment to moment respiratory adjustments. They are relatively insensitive to oxygen but will respond to moderate reductions. Hypoxaemia does, however, sensitize the receptors to carbon dioxide.

EXERCISE

Consider how you are breathing at present. How are your chemoreceptors determining the rate and depth of your breathing?

The pulmonary circulation, and gas exchange

Mixed venous blood enters the heart via the inferior and superior vena cavae, and passes to the lungs via the pulmonary trunk and thence via the right and left pulmonary arteries. The lungs therefore receive the entire output from the right side of the heart, in an adult about 6 litres of blood per minute at rest. The blood vessels divide extensively to eventually form the pulmonary capillaries that pass in close contact with the alveoli of the lung. Blood eventually returns to the left side of the heart via the pulmonary veins.

Like all capillaries, the wall of the pulmonary vessels is just one cell thick. Unlike other capillaries, however, they exude very little fluid into the tissue fluid space. Capillary fluid exchange was described in Chapter 3, where it was noted that the main principle was one of the balance (or imbalance) of the physical forces operating across the capillary membrane. Such forces are the hydrostatic fluid pressure gradient, and the osmotic pressure gradient induced by proteins. In most tissues an imbalance in these forces as blood enters a capillary favours the exudation of water (and salts, etc). This does not occur to the same extent in pulmonary capillaries because the hydrostatic pressure of blood within them is much lower than elsewhere and is, in fact, exceeded by the colloid osmotic pressure due to plasma proteins. As a consequence, the physical forces favour fluid drainage into the capillary, rather than out of it. Pressure in the pulmonary arteries is only of the order of 20/8 mmHg (compared with 120/80 mmHg in the aorta).

Upon entering the lungs the blood is not evenly distributed. The low pulmonary arterial pressure is barely sufficient to force blood against gravity to the top of the lungs (when standing or sitting). This means that much of the blood passes to the lower areas of the lungs, and this is largely responsible for the ventilation/perfusion mismatches that are observed in regions of the lungs (Table 6.1, but also see Box 6.8).

Blood entering the lungs is relatively rich in carbon dioxide having picked it up from the tissues, but it will be deficient in oxygen. Nevertheless, it still contains some oxygen and this has a partial pressure of approximately 5.3 kPa; that of carbon dioxide is approximately 6.0 kPa. On passing through the lungs the blood encounters alveoli where the average gas composition is as was noted earlier. As a consequence:

- oxygen will diffuse into the blood (the alveoli–blood gradient is 13.3– 5.3 = +8.0 kPa), and
- carbon dioxide will diffuse out of blood (the alveoli–blood gradient is 5.3– 6.0 = −0.7 kPa).

Table 6.1 Ventilation/perfusion matching, and mismatching, within normal lungs (shown for an individual in a standing or sitting position)

	Ventilation/ perfusion ratio	Alveolar PO_2 (kPa)	Alveolar PCO_2 (kPa)
Apex of lung	3.3	17.5	3.7
Base of lung	0.63	11.8	5.6
Average for whole lungs	**0.83**	**13.3**	**5.4**

Note
Zonal values between the apex and base of the lungs are not shown, but will contribute to the average values.

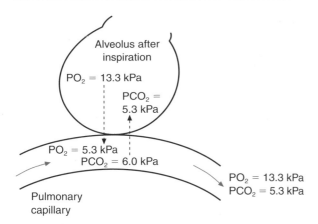

Figure 6.6 **Summary of gas pressures and gas exchange between alveoli and blood**
PO_2 gradient (alveolus–blood) = 13.3 − 5.3 = +8.0 kPa ∴ O_2 diffuses into blood
PCO_2 gradient = 5.3 − 6.0 = −0.7 kPa ∴ CO_2 diffuses out of blood
Gas pressures in blood leaving the alveolus have equilibrated with those of alveolus

Q. Why do you think it is important that the gas pressure gradient for oxygen is much greater than that for carbon dioxide?

The direction of movement of oxygen across the alveolar–capillary membrane is therefore opposite to that of carbon dioxide because the partial pressure gradients of the individual gases are in opposite directions. The situation is summarized in Figure 6.6. Note the small gradient for carbon dioxide. This gas is much more soluble than oxygen and so this gradient is still sufficient to transfer adequate amounts of this gas. Upon leaving the lungs in the pulmonary veins (i.e. = systemic arterial blood) the partial pressures will have equilibrated with those of the alveoli and so the partial pressure of oxygen in blood will now be 13.3 kPa and that of carbon dioxide will be 5.3 kPa.

It must be stressed, however, that normal values for blood gas composition are *average* values for the lungs. The gas composition in alveoli, and in blood leaving these alveoli, varies during a single breath cycle, and also varies between regions of the lung because the relationship between alveolar ventilation and blood perfusion is not consistent. The potential impact of regional differences in ventilation and perfusion within the lungs are explored further in Box 6.8.

EXERCISE

What do the terms hypoxia and hypoxaemia mean? If you are unsure, then refer back to the Introduction of this chapter.

The lung–blood barrier

The barrier between the lung and blood is comprised of the alveolar membrane and the capillary wall (Figure 6.7). The features of this alveolar–capillary membrane have been noted at points in this chapter. Basically:

- the alveolar membrane is one cell thick and the cells are flattened (i.e. squamous) to form an extremely thin structure.
- the capillary wall, or endothelium, is one cell thick and the cells are also flattened to form a very thin membrane.
- physical forces operating within the pulmonary capillaries favour fluid drainage into the blood, rather than out of it as is seen in capillary beds elsewhere. This means that the tissue fluid layer between the alveoli and capillaries is very thin. Lymphatic drainage from the lung interstitium also helps to maintain this thin layer of tissue fluid.
- the huge numbers of alveoli found in the lungs produces an extensive surface area for gas exchange.

One of the common features here is the thinness of the structure. This is important if the solubility of the respiratory gases is taken into account. Both intracellular fluid and tissue fluid are essentially composed of water; oxygen is poorly soluble in water. In fact, even with the partial pressure gradient present between the alveoli and blood, and the thinness of the barrier, it still takes 0.8 seconds for oxygen to cross the barrier and equilibrate with the gas in blood. Fortunately, blood flowing past the alveoli takes slightly longer. For carbon dioxide, being

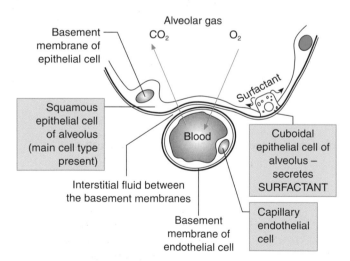

Figure 6.7 Features of the alveolar–capillary membrane

Q. What is the role of surfactant produced by cuboidal epithelial cells?

much more soluble than oxygen in water means that it diffuses more readily from the blood into the alveoli, but the barrier may still be significant in view of the small partial pressure gradient that exists for this gas.

The respiratory system in the perioperative period

Intervention by the theatre team is essential in facilitating the return of effective respiratory function, and hence of blood gas composition, should complications arise during or after surgery. Pre-operative assessment of the patient will provide evidence of pre-existing conditions that might effect the airway, such as tumour, obesity, smoking and anaemia. This will enable appropriately planned perioperative management of the patient by the theatre team to be achieved. However, this is not always possible in emergency situations, and so there are set emergency procedures that are followed by the theatre team.

The previous section illustrated how the relationship between the ventilation of the lungs and their perfusion with blood is essential for blood gas homeostasis. A change in that relationship is the commonest cause of lung-induced hypoxaemia during and after surgery (O'Reilly 2000). To understand the risks introduced by surgery it is therefore necessary to place them into the context of alterations in either ventilation or blood perfusion. It is also necessary to consider how alterations in the features of the lung–blood barrier would influence gas exchange since such changes may also have an impact in the perioperative period.

Box 6.5   Application: related pharmacology for the respiratory system (see also Box 7.1)

Anaesthetics

The respiratory system plays a major part in the uptake and elimination of inhalational anaesthetic agents. Anaesthetic drugs and analgesics may also cause respiratory depression and require clinical intervention.

Inhalational induction agents
The uptake of an inhalational agent into the blood circulation from the alveoli is dependent upon the inspired concentration of the gas, and its solubility in blood.

- *Inspired concentration.* The higher the concentration of the inhalational agent at atmospheric pressure, the more effective it becomes at inducing and maintaining anaesthesia. A maximum concentration of 33 per cent is required to achieve an optimum level of induction and maintain anaesthesia, therefore a lower concentration of gas will produce a longer and possibly more difficult induction.

■ *Solubility in blood*. Inhalational agents of a low solubility only require small amounts to saturate the blood, causing arterial and brain gas tension to rise quickly. Low solubility gases can therefore induce and maintain anaesthesia quickly, and exhibit a rapid recovery as the gas tension is quickly reversed. Agents with a higher solubility, such as halothane, require longer to reach an adequate blood (and hence brain) tension, and recovery may be slower (Carrie *et al.* 1997).

Most inhalational agents depress the respiratory centre of the brain. This results in a decrease in the respiratory minute volume and an increase in the arterial partial pressure of carbon dioxide. However, as noted above, ventilation therapy provides safe airway management and therefore the changes caused by inhalational agents can be quickly and effectively managed. Ventilation therapies are considered in a later section.

Intravenous agents

Most of the intravenous agents given during anaesthesia can cause respiratory depression. Induction agents such as thiopentone decrease the sensitivity of the respiratory centre to carbon dioxide causing respiratory depression and apnoea. Propofol is a non-barbiturate induction agent often used in the patient who is breathing spontaneously. However, it can cause respiratory depression when used in a continuous infusion and careful monitoring of the rate and depth of breathing is necessary.

Analgesics

One of the many side effects of opioid analgesia is respiratory depression (Bailey 1997). Morphine is one of the most commonly used analgesics, and is given in smaller increments to the patient who is breathing spontaneously than to ventilated patients, because of its powerful respiratory effects. Pethidine is a synthetic analgesic which is similar to morphine but has a less sedative effect. Intravenous fentanyl is also a powerful respiratory depressant, but because of its high lipid solubility it has a rapid onset of action. Alfentanil is shorter acting than fentanyl and has a less significant effect on the respiratory system and is often used for spontaneously breathing patients.

Antagonists

Antagonists are drugs that bind to receptors on or within the cells, but do not activate them, and so block or reduce the actions of the active chemicals. They may be used to block the actions of endogenous chemicals, but also may be used to block actions of administered drugs, for example muscle relaxant or opioid analgesics.

The muscle relaxant antagonists neostigmine and glycopyrronium inhibit the action of the enzyme acetylcholinesterase, and so act to slow the breakdown of acetylcholine in the neuromuscular synaptic cleft. In doing so they facilitate transmission, and hence reverse the effect of the muscle relaxants. However, their action will also promote those of acetylcholine elsewhere, where muscle relaxants are not effective. Thus the antagonists will enhance acetylcholine activity at 'muscarinic' and 'nicotinic' receptors in the parasympathetic and sympathetic nerve pathways (see Clancy and McVicar 2002 for a discussion of cholinergic receptors), and so may cause bronchiolar constriction, broncho-secretion, hypotension and increased salivation. Atropine is given as an antagonist to these receptors in order to prevent these side effects from occurring.

Opioid antagonists such as naloxone antagonize any of the opioid analgesics. Naloxone antagonizes both opioid-induced analgesia and respiratory depression equally. It has a 45–90 minute duration of action and can be given in repeated doses if further long-acting opioid drugs have been administered.

Flumazenil is another antagonist, given intravenously, that is used to reverse the effects of benzodiazepine drugs, such as Midazolam, that have anxiolytic, hypnotic, muscle relaxant and anticonvulsant actions (Neal 1997). It has a short duration of action, but should not be regularly employed and used only when necessary.

Perioperative influences on alveolar ventilation: hypoventilation

The discussion in the previous section identifies a number of salient points in relation to maintaining blood gas homeostasis, including:

- establishing appropriate partial pressures of oxygen and carbon dioxide within the alveoli is essential to blood gas composition,
- gas composition within the alveoli is determined by the rate of alveolar ventilation,
- the breathing movements that determine alveolar ventilation are generated by neural activity from the respiratory centres of the brain stem, controlled primarily by input from chemoreceptors centrally and peripherally,
- neural activity from the brain stem promotes muscle contraction of the diaphragm and chest wall,
- low airway resistance and high compliance contribute to the efficiency of this process.

Surgery may influence any of these factors and so promote 'hypoventilation' (hypo- = below normal), a situation in which lung function is inadequate for metabolic needs (Mecca 1999). Thus, inspiration does not promote adequate oxygenation of blood, nor is carbon dioxide in blood sufficiently reduced; this results in hypoxaemia and hypercapnia. Their occurrence should ordinarily promote a homeostatic response to correct the disturbance but the impact of surgery might prevent a normal response, and so they persist. Hypoventilation may arise from a number of causes (summarized in Table 6.2).

EXERCISE

Review your understanding of the terms hypoventilation, hypoxaemia, hypercapnia, dyspnoea, tachypnoea and apnoea.

Table 6.2 **Potential causes of hypoventilation, and the rationale for nursing care in the perioperative period (see also O'Brien 1996)**

Homeostatic failure	Cause	Care
Airway obstruction	Tongue	Mandibular support to maintain airway patency in the unconscious patient.
	Airway compression	Observe for laryngeal oedema, or haematoma in the neck.
	Inhalation of gastric secretions	Reduce risk of vomit aspiration by maintaining nil-by-mouth prior to surgery, or use gastric evacuation.
	Bronchospasm	Observe for signs of airway irritation.
	Accumulation of mucus through cough suppression by analgesics	Facilitate changes in position in post-operative period to reduce risk. Encourage coughing. Use of steam inhalation.
Neurologic/muscle dysfunction	Respiratory depression caused by analgesics or anaesthetics	Encourage breathing movement post-operatively.
	Prolonged effects of muscle relaxants	Check that correct dose of antagonist is administered. Encourage breathing movement post-operatively.
	Post-operative pain	Ensure adequate analgesia. Encourage breathing movements.
Pleural disturbance	Pneumothorax	Care of chest tube inserted for the removal of gas.
	Pleural effusion	Needle aspiration of excess fluid or blood.

Poor neuromuscular response

Anaesthetic and analgesic drugs such as induction agents, opioids and benzo-diazepines may affect the respiratory centre of the brain causing respiratory depression, whilst muscle relaxants will affect the respiratory muscles which may cause apnoea or reduced respiratory effort. If the oxygen saturation falls severely, positive pressure ventilation via a mask and self-inflating bag is likely to be used by a skilled practitioner, though if the oxygen saturation continues to fall, tracheal intubation should be considered (see later section entitled 'Ventilation therapy as a homeostatic mechanism').

If consciousness has returned but there has been incomplete reversal of the muscle relaxant, the patient may be extremely distressed; this may present with unco-ordinated limb movements and associated tachycardia and hypertension. The correct antagonist may need to be administered (see Box 6.5). The perioperative practitioner should also provide reassurance and an encouragement to breathe.

Pain

Post-operative pain may affect the patient's breathing movements and so lead to hypoventilation and hypoxaemia. Using modern anaesthetics the belief is that the prevention of pain prior to the painful stimulus will result in less pain, and so pain relief may be given pre-operatively as part of the patient's pre-medication, intraoperatively and post-operatively, thus ensuring optimum pain relief for the patient. However, post-operative pain may still occur and the respiratory effort of the patient may be affected. Adequate pain relief is essential to facilitate deep breathing, although the use of opioid analgesia may induce respiratory depression. The patient's oxygen saturation should be monitored and oxygen therapy may be required for several days post-operatively.

Pleural dysfunction

Pneumothorax may occur when there has been trauma or surgery to the chest, or through insertion of central venous lines via the subclavian or jugular route, or where patients with predisposing lung disease have required high pressure mechanical ventilation (Ares and Fein 1995). Air entering the pleural space prevents normal lung inflation, causing lung collapse; subsequently lung compression and alteration in the venous return to the heart occurs. The patient may develop dyspnoea or tachypnoea. An underwater sealed chest drain must be inserted to allow air to escape and the lung to re-inflate. It is important that the perioperative practitioner observes the drain for any signs of blood and or fluid loss. Other observations include ensuring the the distal end of the drain remains under water as this ensures lung inflation and subsequent sealing of the leak. These patients are nursed in the sitting position wherever possible and close observation of their oxygen saturation and breathing effort is essential. Oxygen therapy may be necessary for several days post-operatively.

Airway obstruction through compression, bronchospasm, mucus or inflammation

Airway obstruction can occur at any time during the perioperative period. It may be caused by pre-medication and anaesthetic drugs, trauma or surgery to the airway, anaphylaxis, bronchospasm or accumulation of mucus in the airway.

The tongue can be responsible for airway obstruction: the muscles of the throat lose their muscular tone, or the soft palate, tongue and epiglottis fall against the posterior pharyngeal wall. This causes the walls of the throat to collapse during inspiration and obstructs the airway. Mandibular support is required to maintain the airway (see Figure 6.8).

Airway compression is possible as a result of laryngeal oedema or tracheal compression due to post-operative haemorrhage; for example following neck surgery. The patient must be closely observed for signs of oedema and haemorrhage; if haemorrhage occurs, exploratory/corrective surgery may be necessary. It is extremely important that the perioperative practitioner has a suture or skin staple remover available during the post-operative period, when caring for patients who have had surgery which might compromise the upper airway, e.g. thyroidectomy.

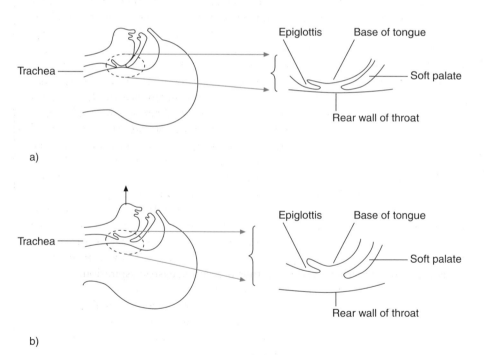

Figure 6.8 Mandibular manipulation to maintain an open airway
a   Obstruction of the airway by oropharyngeal features during anaesthesia
b   Removing airway obstruction by application of chin lift.

Q. What is the usual role of the epiglottis?

Inhalation of gastric contents through aspiration (see Box 6.6), or of blood or mucus, presents a serious risk to the patient's airway and subsequent recovery. Pre-operative fasting can reduce the risk of inhalation of gastric contents. Patients who are identified as being 'at risk' may be treated pre-operatively with antacids to reduce gastric acidity; acid secretion may be reduced by administration of a histamine (H_2) antagonist, and a rapid sequence induction of anaesthesia is used.

Box 6.6 Application: gastric aspiration

One factor of particular concern during and after surgery is the possibility of aspiration of gastric contents, as a consequence of the actions of general anaesthetic which relax the cardiac sphincter of the stomach and act directly on the emetic (vomiting) centres of the brain stem (Chapter 7).

Aspiration of gastric contents causes inflammation and bronchospasm, which increase airway resistance, pulmonary oedema and a risk of physical damage to the alveolar-capillary membrane, leading to intra-alveolar bleeding (Quinn 1998). The progression of the effects of the gastric acid on the airways means that the problem persists into the post-surgical period. The presence of pulmonary oedema makes oxygen therapy ineffective (see later in this chapter) and gastric aspiration is therefore a very serious complication with a high risk of fatality. Collectively, the condition and its symptoms are referred to as aspiration pneumonitis, or Mendelson's syndrome.

Prior to elective surgery the patient is normally starved to ensure that the stomach is free of undigested food (see section entitled 'Pre-operative influences on water balance' in Chapter 3). The maintenance of the patient's airway is absolutely essential and the use of a cuffed endotracheal tube, once inflated, protects the airway. Other types of airway maintenance can be used and these are dependent on the type of surgery being performed and the physical condition of the patient. Gastric aspiration is prevented on induction of anaesthesia by compressing the trachea prior to placement of the endotracheal tube. To do this, the anaesthetic assistant applies finger pressure to the cricoid cartilage of the trachea (Bryant and Tingen 1999). This cartilage is found at the base of the larynx (at the level of the C6 vertebra) and is the only tracheal cartilage that forms a complete circle. Applying pressure to the cricoid compresses the oesophagus between the posterior aspect of the cartilage and the underlying vertebrae, thus preventing gastric aspiration.

The manoeuvre is especially used in emergency situations. In such situations, adequate pre-operative starving is not always possible and so appropriate action must be taken. Increased pressure on the stomach, for example in a pregnant woman undergoing a caesarean section, also increases the likelihood of aspiration.

A nasogastric or orogastric tube may also be used to aspirate liquid stomach contents prior to and during surgery. However, if left in they can cause the cardiac sphincter of the stomach to be less competent, and are not guaranteed to empty the stomach.

EXERCISE

In which part of the airways would you expect bronchospasm to occur? (Clue: where is smooth muscle found?)

Bronchospasm commonly occurs as a result of an irritant to the lungs, e.g. a response to an allergen, asthma, smoking or due to respiratory infection. During anaesthesia it may be induced by the sudden inspiration of too high a concentration of volatile anaesthetic agent, or as a result of surgical stimulus when the level of anaesthesia is too light. The bronchospasm can be resolved either by removing the stimulus, deepening the level of anaesthesia, increasing the level of inspired oxygen concentration and if necessary the administration of bronchodilators and steroids. Close observation of the airway is essential for early detection of airway irritation, as this allows rapid and effective intervention by the theatre team.

Accumulation of secretions in the lungs during the perioperative period can occur, possibly as a result of suppression of the cough reflex by analgesics or through pain from the surgical incision. Upper abdominal incisions in particular can cause compressional collapse of the lungs and pain from the surgical incision

Box 6.7   Application: hyperventilation

The text identifies 'hypoventilation' as a breathing pattern that is inadequate for the metabolic needs of the body. 'Hyperventilation' is the opposite, in which breathing is in excess of body needs. The effect is readily demonstrated: take a deep breath, breathe out maximally and then rapidly take another deep breath (it is not advisable to do this for more than just a small number of breaths). You should feel a little dizzy as the large volume of air breathed in produces a greater than normal reduction in blood carbon dioxide concentration. The dizziness arises because of a reduction in blood flow to the brain as a result of the effect of the deeper breath to reduce the carbon dioxide content of blood (in a sense, hyperventilating lungs 'wash out' more carbon dioxide than normal). Lowering the carbon dioxide content of blood in this way also induces a respiratory alkalosis since the generation of acidity from the gas is reduced. The oxygen content of blood is little changed during hyperventilation as blood is normally almost saturated with oxygen anyway.

Hyperventilation may be observed in anxiety or when someone is in pain. Healthcare professionals should be aware of the possible consequences and take steps to reassure the patient, or reduce pain, in order to reduce the hyperventilation.

EXERCISE

Suggest why we don't normally feel dizzy when we take deeper breaths during moderate exercise.

can make breathing shallow and coughing ineffective. Post-operatively, the patient should be sat up as soon as possible and coughing encouraged. Oxygen therapy may be required for several days post-operatively, as well as physiotherapy and possibly drugs such as bronchodilators and antibiotics.

The delivery of anaesthetic gases, oxygen, nitrous oxide and volatile agents will also be affected if there is an airway obstruction. A reduction in the delivery of the anaesthetic gases can lead to an increase in the level of consciousness, awareness, movement, coughing or laryngeal spasm.

Perioperative influences on pulmonary blood supply: pulmonary embolism

The presence of an embolism is a major cause of reduced pulmonary blood supply in the perioperative period, and increases the reliance upon remaining functioning alveoli. The lungs are particularly susceptible to emboli because of their position: pulmonary capillaries are the first capillary bed encountered by blood after returning to the heart from the tissues.

Pulmonary embolism (Reid 1999; Epley 2000) is caused by:

- a fat embolus released from fat-containing tissues, such as bone marrow,
- a blood embolus dislodged from a blood clot,
- an air embolus introduced into a vein, or via rupture of alveoli.

Fat emboli are relatively common, particularly where there has been bone fracture (bone marrow has a high fat component). However, the main risk after surgery is generally from the formation of blood emboli, and so it is important to take measures to prevent their occurrence (Epley 2000). Leg exercises and early ambulation will help to prevent venous stasis and the development of a peripheral blood clot, and so reduce the risk of a blood embolus. Prophylactic anticoagulants may also be used.

Disseminated intravascular coagulation (DIC) is another cause of blood emboli within the lungs (and other tissues). DIC arises when systemic hypoxia (for example, following profound hypotension or haemorrhagic shock) causes damage to and a roughening of the endothelium of blood vessel walls, and the release of tissue thromboplastin from damaged cells (Rutherford 1996). The roughened vessel walls trigger platelets to initiate the intrinsic clotting process, whilst the thromboplastin initiates the extrinsic process (see Chapter 5). The systemic nature of the hypoxia means that clotting will be widespread, exacerbating the lack of circulation through the lungs and other tissues (Atassi and Harris 2001). DIC, therefore, is lifethreatening. Paradoxically, DIC also increases the risk of haemorrhage. This is because the widespread activation of the clotting cascade removes the clotting factors from plasma, making further clotting less likely should tissue trauma occur.

Pulmonary emboli may break up and disappear with time, though the lysis of a blood embolus can be hastened by the use of fibrinolytic drugs, or rapid-acting anticoagulants in DIC. Supplemental oxygen (see 'Ventilation therapy as a homeostatic mechanism', p. 205) is used to raise alveolar oxygen pressure and promote oxygen uptake in functioning alveoli, in order to provide compensation for nonfunctioning alveoli.

Box 6.8   Application: surgery and the ventilation/perfusion ratio

Ordinarily, total pulmonary ventilation and the rate of blood perfusion of the lungs are almost matched (in an adult at rest about 5–6 litres per minute and 6–7 litres per minute, respectively) and this facilitates the process of gas exchange in the alveoli. Although there is a reasonable matching of whole lung ventilation and perfusion, there is extensive regional variation within the lungs as a consequence of uneven ventilation and blood distribution (Table 6.1). Obviously, blood draining from the lungs as a whole, and returning to the heart into systemic circulation, will be a mixture of blood from the different regions of the lungs. The gas composition of the blood therefore reflects the net effect of these regional differences, and represents an average gas exchange for the lungs as a whole.

Regional disturbances in the ventilation–perfusion ratio arising from surgery will alter gas exchange in the affected areas and so promote an alteration in the net composition of blood leaving the lungs.

- For example (Table 6.1), upon sitting or standing, at the apex of the lung the alveoli are relatively better ventilated than they are perfused with blood. This relatively excessive ventilation will only oxygenate blood as normal since blood is already almost fully saturated with oxygen during normal ventilation. However, carbon dioxide will be removed more efficiently (since the alveoli are in effect being hyperventilated – see Box 6.7).

  A potential problem is that a high ventilation–perfusion ratio arising elsewhere contributes a 'physiological' dead space. This is especially the case if there is insufficient blood to produce significant gas exchange since the ventilation is in a sense wasted. The higher-than-average partial pressure of oxygen in such alveoli is then of little or no benefit. A lack of blood supply, for example by the presence of an embolus, therefore promotes a 'dead space effect' as there is reduced gas exchange overall by the lung and hence a net reduction in the oxygen content of blood leaving the lung.

- At the base of the lung (Table 6.1) the alveoli are relatively better perfused than they are ventilated. These alveoli therefore could be viewed as being hypoventilated and so blood leaving this area will not be oxygenated fully and will also retain more carbon dioxide. In health, ventilation of the upper areas of the lung compensates for the poor gas exchange at the lung base. However, if other parts of the lung also become hypoventilated there will be a resultant reduction in the partial pressure of oxygen in blood leaving the lungs. This may be considered as producing a 'shunt effect' because it is as though some blood has missed the lungs entirely, and been shunted from the right side of the heart directly to the left. Shunt effects are considered relative to blood gas composition produced should a *complete* right–left shunt have occurred and the greater the effect (5 per cent, 10 per cent, etc.) the more significant the systemic hypoxaemia.

Perioperative influences on the alveolar–capillary membrane: pulmonary oedema

There are two general ways in which the barrier to oxygen diffusion may be increased:

■ fibrosis of the alveolar–capillary membrane is a possible long-term complication of respiratory failure leading to a loss of elasticity and a decreased vital capacity, and deteriorating lung function.

■ excess tissue fluid and/or fluid within the alveoli (pulmonary oedema).

There are a number of causes of pulmonary oedema (Kenny 1997), a condition that can arise very quickly and be fatal (Arieff 1999; Seigh 1999). First, tissue and alveolar fluid may accumulate when the physical forces operating across the capillary wall are disturbed, for example by pulmonary hypertension. In surgery, an increased alveolar–capillary permeability induced by inhaled gases or other factors (see 'Acute respiratory failure', p. 204) will also promote pulmonary oedema as proteins leak out of the plasma and into alveoli, thus disturbing the balance between hydrostatic and colloid (protein) osmotic pressure.

Second, pulmonary oedema may arise from an accumulation of fluid as part of an inflammatory process. Biochemical mediators of inflammation are produced by certain cells of the immune system in response to the presence of irritants (e.g. gastric aspiration, Box 6.6), toxins or microorganisms. Immune responses to infection, and the endotoxins produced by bacteria, may also damage the alveolar–capillary membrane, thus exacerbating any oedema and initiating fibrosis. The accumulation of secretions within the lungs following surgery as a consequence of decreased movement, fluid overload, poor respiratory effort or in response to anaesthetic gases provides an environment in which microorganisms can thrive, and so there is a risk of pneumonia.

Pneumonia is caused by bacteria or viruses. Many of the causative organisms are present within the oropharynx in health but they are not normally pathogenic because of the effectiveness of mucus trapping and removal by mucociliary clearance, the cough reflex and of macrophage activity within the alveoli. Viral pneumonia causes destruction of ciliated cells within the airways and mucus production is increased; both actions increase the chance of a secondary bacterial infection. Viral pneumonia is self-limiting, whereas bacteria will normally respond to appropriate antibiotics.

Whatever the cause, the presence of pulmonary oedema provides a substantial barrier to the diffusion of oxygen, because oxygen is poorly soluble in water. Under these circumstances, the partial pressure of oxygen in alveoli may be normal or near normal (depending upon the extent of changes in airway resistance) but will not be sufficient to drive enough oxygen across the additional fluid barrier. This results in hypoxaemia.

Supplemental oxygen should be provided to elevate the alveolar partial pressure of oxygen and thus increase the pressure gradient between alveoli and blood in order to facilitate diffusion (see 'Ventilation therapy as a homeostatic mechanism', p. 205). Oxygen therapy is not immensely effective, however, because the low solubility of the gas will still be a limiting factor in its diffusion across the layer of exudate. Preventing pneumonia from developing is therefore preferable and an important role of the nurse (Reed 1996). Encouraging deep breathing using 'incentive spirometry', coughing, position changing and ambulation are important aspects in the prevention of pneumonia, and in its treatment.

EXERCISE

What is 'incentive spirometry'?

Acute respiratory failure

Individually, the alterations to lung function identified in this section as potential perioperative risks are problematic. However, some disturbances may occur simultaneously and so the difficulties are exacerbated. 'Acute respiratory failure' is an example of cumulative problems. Its most severe form is called the 'adult respiratory distress syndrome' (ARDS) and has a very high mortality rate despite active intervention (Cutler 1996; Sachdeva and Guntupalli 1997). Acute respiratory failure may be observed after trauma, including surgery.

The aetiology of post-surgical respiratory failure is poorly understood. Risk factors for its development include smoking, pre-existing lung disease, cardiac problems, chronic kidney or liver pathologies and infection (Bukowski and Peters 1994; Sadikot and Christman 1999). Surgery of the thorax or abdomen carries a high risk of precipitating acute respiratory failure, presumably because the trauma involved is more severe and hence is a greater stressor (Chapter 7).

The changes observed in the lungs are those of a large inflammatory response, and include:

■ airway inflammation, leading to obstruction and hypoventilation. Atelectasis may occur.
■ the secretion of exudates by inflamed tissue, resulting in pulmonary oedema.
■ the exudation of fluid from pulmonary capillaries into the alveoli as a consequence of an elevated permeability of the alveolar–capillary membrane, and the leakage of plasma proteins into the alveoli. This latter effect disturbs the balance of forces that govern fluid exchange at capillary level and promote the further accumulation of oedematous fluid within the alveoli.

Respiratory failure is characterized, therefore, by a combination of some of those factors identified earlier as causes of hypoxaemia. This combination of pulmonary oedema with a decreased ventilation/perfusion ratio causes diagnostic changes:

■ a severe hypoxaemia ($PaO_2 < 6.6$ kPa; normal $= 13.3$ kPa),
■ hypercapnia ($PaCO_2 > 6.6$ kPa; normal $= 5.4$ kPa),
■ acidosis (pH < 7.25; normal $= 7.35–7.45$).

It has already been noted that the management of blood gas composition in the presence of pulmonary oedema is difficult; respiratory failure after surgery is therefore a serious complication.

Frequent turning and early ambulation will reduce the risk of atelectasis and the accumulation of secretions. Incentive spirometry can also be used to encourage progressively improved tidal volumes. This helps to improve lung ventilation and also loosens secretions. Steroids may be used to reduce the inflammation that is responsible for the problem, but steroid therapy has not proved universally successful. Oxygen therapy and antibiotics may also be used.

Ventilation therapy as a homeostatic mechanism

Effective airway management during the perioperative phase is essential for the maintenance of respiratory homeostasis, by ensuring adequate delivery of oxygen and anaesthetic gases as well as the removal of carbon dioxide. Patients are usually able to maintain their own airway when they are having local or regional procedures performed or, for example, when receiving sedation for pain relief in labour or dental surgery. The effectiveness can alter and close observation of the patient is essential. Any alteration in the patient's breathing pattern might be significant (see Figure 6.9); for example, stridor and cyanosis indicate airway obstruction. The monitoring of vital signs is also important; a fall in oxygen saturation, indicated by the pulse oximeter and changes in heart rate and electrocardiogram reading, provide an indication of respiratory insufficiency. However, these changes tend to arise only after the early clinical signs have been observed and so should be preventable.

Patients who are experiencing difficulty in maintaining respiratory function will receive ventilation therapy to facilitate gas exchange, and so promote a normalization of blood gas composition. Ventilation therapy during the perioperative phase can be achieved in different ways, from basic oxygen therapy in the patient breathing spontaneously to mechanical ventilation where independent breathing is not possible.

Oxygen therapy

Oxygen therapy for patients who can breathe spontaneously, but have inadequate alveolar ventilation, may be delivered via face mask or nasal cannula (Oh 1997; Vines *et al.* 2000). The patient's clinical condition and the type of mask or cannula used will determine the rate of flow.

Oxygen masks are designed to give a set percentage of oxygen; a flow of 4 litres per minute will provide an oxygen percentage of 35 per cent, whilst a flow of 10 litres per minute will provide an oxygen percentage of 60 per cent. These percentages are in excess of that in air and raise the partial pressure of oxygen accordingly (Sykes 1995). For example, an oxygen percentage of 60 per cent in air yields a partial pressure of oxygen of about 60 kPa, compared with about 21 kPa in air. Nasal cannulae are not as effective as oxygen masks because the patient may also breathe air through the mouth. A flow rate of 2–3 litres per minute will only provide an oxygen percentage of about 25–28 per cent (a partial pressure of oxygen of about 25–28 kPa) but this is still in excess of that found in air.

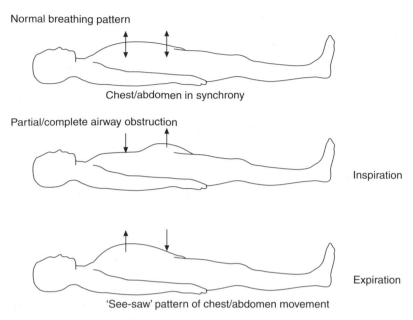

Normal breathing pattern

Chest/abdomen in synchrony

Partial/complete airway obstruction

Inspiration

Expiration

'See-saw' pattern of chest/abdomen movement

Figure 6.9 **Normal and abnormal breathing patterns**

Q. How does the exaggerated abdominal movement help lung ventilation when the airway is partially blocked?

Alveolar ventilation is not improved by these methods of ventilation, but the enriched mixture raises the partial pressure of oxygen within the alveoli and so facilitates uptake. A little carbon dioxide is normally added to the inhalant mixture to prevent disturbances in this gas, and the improvement in the alveolar oxygen is mainly at the expense of nitrogen, the most prevalent gas in air. Carbon dioxide excretion, therefore, is not substantially improved by this method.

EXERCISE

Why can pure oxygen not be administered?

When the patient is anaesthetized but breathing spontaneously, the airway can be maintained by using a face mask and jaw support; or an oral airway might also be employed. A laryngeal mask airway is effective in maintaining oxygenation. It can be attached to an anaesthetic circuit with a reservoir bag, which can be used as another monitoring system since the movements of the reservoir bag should reflect respiratory effort by the patient (note: only if there is adequate gas flow into the system!). A gas analyser incorporated into the breathing circuit provides for measurements of inspired and expired gas concentrations, and gas flow and volumes to be assessed. This provides evidence of the patency of the airway and the adequacy of ventilation as the inspired and expired carbon dioxide levels can be ascertained (Morton 1997).

In some patients, it may be necessary to maintain positive pressure within the lungs during the breathing cycle. This is referred to as Continuous Positive Airway Pressure (CPAP).[1] The pressure is applied via an endotracheal tube, mask or nasal prongs, and so increases the patency of alveoli and helps to prevent their collapse. It may also help to redistribute fluid into the tissue fluid space from the alveoli. In these ways, CPAP improves ventilation/perfusion matching, and reduces any alveolar membrane problems arising from fluid accumulation. The risk is that the elevated pressure may induce barotrauma (baro- = pressure) by decreasing the output to the lungs from the right side of the heart (and subsequently cardiac output from the left side). Hyperinflation also decreases the compliance of the lungs, making them harder to inflate (i.e. the work of breathing is increased), and increases the risk of pneumothorax occurring.

Mechanical ventilation therapy

Mechanical ventilation therapy is used when an individual's spontaneous breathing is inadequate (Turner et al. 1997). It may become necessary during the perioperative period when muscle relaxant drugs have been used, or when respiratory movements are severely reduced, for example in cases of trauma where the patient is unable to protect their own airway (Tan and Oh 1997).

In Intermittent Positive Pressure Ventilation (IPPV), an enriched gas mixture is inhaled at a pressure greater than atmospheric and thus the alveoli are ventilated. As the term IPPV implies, this mode of ventilation does not continuously apply positive pressure. The administration of muscle relaxants may be required to ensure patient compliance. The procedure also reduces the respiratory effort required from the patient. Exhalation is passive, as normal, and airway pressure therefore decreases during expiration to the atmospheric pressure or slightly below it.

The equipment may control the volume of air provided (with a potential risk of excessive airway pressures if resistance is high) or control the pressure (though the volume of air delivered may vary). Thus, IPPV requires close monitoring of both pressure and volume of air delivery (Box 6.9).

EXERCISE

What are the specific indications for tracheal intubation in general anaesthesia?

[1] Bi-Positive Airway Pressure (BiPAP) is a modification of CPAP that is used in intensive care and should not be confused with CPAP. In BiPAP two airway pressures are applied, with synchronization during the breathing cycle. It too ensures a positive end-expiration pressure (PEEP) but it also allows a reduction in pressure during the expiration (though a positive pressure is still maintained) and this helps to reduce the risk of barotrauma and decreased compliance. The pressure is increased once more during inspiration, and this helps to inflate the alveoli.

> ### Box 6.9 Application: adjustment of mechanical ventilators
>
> Mechanical ventilation may be applied in a variety of ways but a basic principle is that a ventilator forces gas into the lungs during the inspiratory phase of a breathing cycle, but exhalation is passive. The ventilator therefore must terminate inspiration at an appropriate point, having delivered an adequate tidal volume. Terminating inspiration is achieved either by pressure-cycling, or time-cycling.
>
> #### Pressure-cycling
>
> Pressure-cycled ventilators terminate inspiration when a pre-set pressure in the circuit is achieved. One potential difficulty with this method is that a rapid rise in pressure will terminate inspiration early and so deliver an inadequate volume of gas. This might be caused by:
>
> - elevated airway resistance that prevents the usual flow of gas into the lungs. The pressure upstream of the resistance will then rise more quickly.
> - reduced lung compliance (i.e. elasticity) that prevents normal expansion of the lungs. The reduced lung expansion will make pressure within the lungs rise rapidly during inspiration.
>
> Pressure-cycled ventilation therefore may not maintain a constant tidal volume, and hence alveolar ventilation may be poorly controlled.
>
> #### Time-cycling
>
> Time-cycled ventilators terminate inspiration after a pre-set time interval. The tidal volume that is delivered will depend upon the duration of the inspiration, and also on the gas flow rate during this time (which is unlikely to remain constant due to pressure change within the circuit). Pressure changes could therefore have a significant effect on the volume of gas that is delivered, and hence on alveolar ventilation.

Summary

- Blood gas homeostasis is a vital part of the process of maintaining tissue oxygenation, and in preventing acidosis arising from carbon dioxide accumulation.
- The partial pressures of respiratory gases in arterial blood reflect those of the gases within the lung alveoli during the breathing cycle, but should be viewed as being representative of average alveolar composition since there is regional variation within the lungs.

■ There is a need, therefore, for homeostatic processes to control lung function if tissue functions elsewhere are to be supported.

■ The control of lung function is very precise, but it is susceptible to extrinsic factors.

■ Inadequate alveolar ventilation, changes in the regional distribution of ventilation or blood flow, and alterations to the alveolar–capillary membrane across which the gases must diffuse result in a failure to maintain blood gas homeostasis. Correcting hypoxaemia is generally of more immediate concern in the perioperative period, although carbon dioxide content must also be monitored because of its link with acidosis.

■ Causes of poor respiratory function in the perioperative period include:
  – depressant effects of anaesthesia.
  – influence of anxiety or pain to produce over-breathing, i.e. hyperventilation.
  – influence of thoracic pain possibly to restrict breathing movement.
  – depressant actions of opioid analgesics.
  – complications of the surgical process, e.g. gastric aspiration, respiratory failure.

■ It is important that perioperative staff are aware of the risk of respiratory complication during and after surgery, and of the difficulties in providing effective intervention, including ventilation therapy.

■ Risk reduction and the need for monitoring should be a primary feature of care planning and delivery.

■ Ventilation therapies provide a means of maintaining or improving alveolar ventilation and gas exchange. Alveolar gas composition may be improved using oxygen-enriched air, or assisted ventilation may be used to support spontaneous breathing or even to replace it. Positive pressure may be applied to maintain patency of the airways and alveoli, but the method does have risks. It is important that perioperative professionals are aware of the basis of ventilation therapy, the potential risks, and the need for careful monitoring.

Bibliography

Ares, C.A. and Fein, A.M. (1995) Pneumothorax. *Emergency Medicine* 27(12): 62–70.

Arieff, A.I. (1999) Fatal postoperative pulmonary edema: pathogenesis and literature review. *Chest* 115(5): 1371–7.

Ashurst, S. (1997) Nursing care of the mechanically ventilated patient in ITU. *British Journal of Nursing* 6(8): 447–54.

Atassi, K.A. and Harris, M.L. (2001) Disseminated intravascular coagulation. *Nursing* 31(3): 64.

Bailey, P.L. (1997) Opioid-induced respiratory depression. *Current Reviews for Perianaesthesia Nurses* 19(17): 171–80.

British National Formulary (2002) *British National Formulary* (41). London: BMA/Royal Pharmaceutical Society.

Bryant, A. and Tingen, M.S. (1999) The use of cricoid pressure during emergency intubation. *Journal of Emergency Nursing* 25(4): 283–4.

Bukowski, D.M. and Peters, J.I. (1994) Acute respiratory failure: diagnosis and management. *Hospital Medicine* 30(12): 52–70.

Carrie, L.E.S., Simpson, P.J. and Popat, M.T. (1997) *Understanding Anaesthesia, Third Edition*. Oxford: Butterworth Heinemann.

Clancy, J. and McVicar, A.J. (2002) *Physiology and Anatomy: a Homeostatic Approach, Second Edition*: London: Arnold.

Cutler, R. (1996) Acute respiratory distress syndrome: an overview. *Intensive and Critical Care Nursing* 12(6): 316–26.

Epley, D. (2000) Pulmonary emboli risk reduction. *Journal of Vascular Nursing* 18(2): 61–70.

Griffiths, R. (1999a) Anaesthesia: airway management. *British Journal of Perioperative Nursing* 9(10): 480–3.

Griffiths, R. (1999b) Anaesthesia: breathing management. *British Journal of Perioperative Nursing* 9(11): 537–9.

Griffiths, R. (2000) Breathing circuits and their uses. *British Journal of Perioperative Nursing* 10(1): 55–9.

Kenny, M.F. (1997) Acute pulmonary edema. *Nursing* 27(11): 33.

Maxson, J.H. (2000) Management of disseminated intravascular coagulation. *Critical Care Nursing Clinics of North America* 12(3): 341–52.

Mecca, R.S. (1999) Postoperative hypercarbia. *Current Reviews for Perianesthesia Nurses* 21(10): 90–100.

Morton, N.S. (1997) *Assisting the Anaesthetist*. Oxford: Oxford University Press.

Moyle, J.B., Hahn, C.E.W. and Adams, A.P. (1998) *Pulse Oximetry*. London: BMJ Books.

Neal, M.J. (1997) *Medical Pharmacology at a Glance, Third Edition*. Oxford: Blackwell Science.

O'Brien, D.D. (1996) The perioperative nurse in the postanesthesia care unit, in *Perioperative Nursing Care Planning, Second Edition*, St Louis: Mosby, pp. 496 and 591.

Oh, T.E. (1997) Oxygen therapy, in *Intensive Care Manual, Fourth Edition*, Oxford: Butterworth Heinmann, pp. 209–16.

O'Reilly, D. (2000) Adult hypoxemia in the perioperative period: a review of the literature. *British Journal of Perioperative Nursing* 10(4): 204–12.

Quinn, C.E. (1998) Gastric aspiration. *Emergency Medicine* 30(9): 97–104.

Reed, C. (1996) Care of postoperative patients with pulmonary edema. *Journal of Perianesthesia Nursing* 11(3): 164–9.

Reid, E. (1999) Pulmonary embolism: an overview of treatment and nursing issues. *British Journal of Nursing* 8(20): 1373–8.

Rutherford, I.A. (1996) Haemostasis and disseminated intravascular coagulation. *Intensive and Critical Care Nursing* 12(3): 161–7.

Sachdeva, R.C. and Guntupalli, K.K. (1997) Acute respiratory distress syndrome. *Critical Care Clinics* 13(3): 503–21.

Sadikot, R.T. and Christman, J.W. (1999) ARDS: how and when does it develop? Early identification of patients at risk may be the key. *Journal of Respiratory Diseases* 20(6): 438–44.

Seigh, P.J. (1999) Emergency! Pulmonary oedema: will you have to intubate? *American Journal of Nursing* 99(12): 43.

Sykes, K. (1995) *Respiratory Support*. London: British Medical Journal Publishing Group.

Tan, I.K.S. and Oh, T.E. (1997) Mechanical ventilation support, in *Intensive Care Manual*, T.E. Oh (ed.), Butterworth Heinemann, pp. 246–55.

Turner, P., Glass, C. and Grap, M.J. (1997) Care of the patient requiring mechanical ventilation. *Medical Surgical Nursing* 6(2): 68–94.

Vines, D.L., Shelledy, D.C. and Peters, J. (2000) Current respiratory care, Part 1: oxygen therapy, oximetry, bronchial hygiene. *Journal of Critical Illness* 15(9): 507–10.

Warner, M.E. (1997) Ambulatory surgery. Risks and outcomes of perioperative pulmonary aspiration. *Journal of Perianesthesia Nursing* 12(5): 352–7.

Chapter 7

Anaesthesia, stress and surgery

Introduction

Generally speaking, stress is considered to arise as a consequence of the interaction with one's external environment, entailing a conscious or subconscious cognitive appraisal of the situation (Clancy and McVicar 2002, Chapter 22). Indicators of stress arise when the individual's perceived ability to meet the perceived demand is inadequate, and so that demand becomes a distressor.

Whilst this view of stress could be applied to someone anticipating surgery, it does not immediately lend itself to explaining the physiological responses that may arise during surgery, yet these are similar to a 'classic' stress response in many respects. To understand how this can be so, it is necessary to place stress responses into context, and so this section continues with a conventional view of the physical responses to stress by considering the 'General Adaptation Syndrome', first proposed by Hans Selye in 1956.

The General Adaptation Syndrome

If stress indicators normally relate to perceptions, this raises the question as to how cognitive processes can have such a profound influence on an individual's physiology. The answer lies within the two co-ordinating systems that are fundamental to homeostatic control: the autonomic nervous system and the endocrine (hormonal) system (Figure 7.1). The neural link arises from connections between the higher centres of the brain and the autonomic nerves, especially those of the sympathetic division. The actions of sympathetic nerves may be supported by the release of catecholamine hormones from the adrenal glands.

The hormonal link especially involves secretions of the anterior pituitary gland, controlled by the hypothalamus and thus influenced by higher centres.

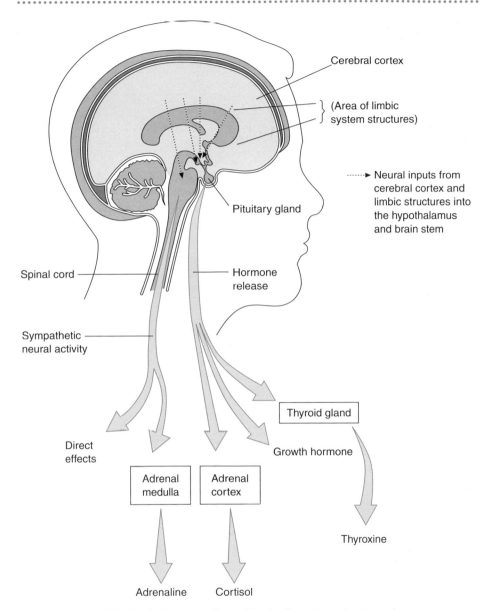

Figure 7.1 'Mind–body' links. An outline of the biological mechanisms that promote stress responses

Q. Which hormone is produced by the adrenal cortex and which by the adrenal medulla?

Details of hormonal actions are provided later, but basically the hormones involved are:

- *adrenocorticotropin* (or adrenocorticotropic hormone; ACTH) secretion leads to the release of corticosteroid hormones, especially *cortisol*, from the adrenal cortex. Cortisol is a hormone that influences metabolism.
- *growth hormone* secretion. This hormone has direct metabolic actions on body tissues.
- *thyrotropin* (or thyroid-stimulating hormone; TSH) secretion leads to the release of *thyroxine* from the thyroid gland. Thyroxine is also a metabolic hormone.

EXERCISE

Review:

- the structure of the pituitary gland, and its division into anterior and posterior parts, and
- the hormones produced by each part.

How is the hypothalamus involved in the secretion of hormones by the pituitary gland?

Both systems mediate the stress response. Initial descriptions of the biological responses to stressors are attributed to the work of Selye (1956), who proposed that stress invokes a series of responses which he collectively referred to as a 'General Adaptation Syndrome' (GAS). Although the GAS can be criticized from various aspects, notably the sequencing of events, the responses it describes are identifiable in the patient undergoing surgery. The principles of the GAS therefore provide a useful means of introducing these responses, but the reader should bear in mind that the changes it describes, especially the hormonal responses, may occur simultaneously.

Selye identified three phases (Figure 7.2):

- An 'alarm' phase. It is the alarm phase that is characterized by stimulation of the sympathetic division of the autonomic nervous system, and by the release of the catecholamine hormones adrenaline and noradrenaline (called epinephrine and norepinephrine respectively in the USA). Selye viewed this as being anticipatory of a threat and the necessity of taking action through promotion of the 'fear, fight, flight' response (Table 7.1). He suggested that the phase is transient and the individual soon passes into the next phase.
- A 'resistance' phase. The resistance phase is characterized by metabolic changes that were initiated by sympathetic nerve activation in the alarm phase, and maintained by the hormones cortisol, growth hormone and thyroxine. Indeed, cortisol is sometimes referred to as the 'hormone of stress' since individuals who are unable to produce it in sufficient quantities adapt very poorly to stressful situations. The actions of cortisol and growth

Table 7.1 Influence of sympathetic nerve activity (and adrenaline) in the 'fear, fight, flight' response. The significance of the action is indicated in *italics*

Tissue/organ	Sympathetic innervation (and adrenaline)
Heart	Systolic contraction increased, with greater force of contraction and increased pulse rate. *Elevates cardiac output; raises blood pressure.*
Blood vessels	Selective vasoconstriction and vasodilation are induced. *Raise blood pressure and redistribute blood to active tissues.*
Sweat glands	Sweat production is increased. *Helps to dissipate excess heat generated by increased metabolism.*
Salivary glands	Salivation is reduced. *Prevents excess being drawn into the lungs during inhalation.*
Lungs	Bronchodilation is induced that lowers airway resistance. *Facilitates alveolar ventilation.*
Gastrointestinal tract	Blood from the tract is diverted to active tissues. Motility is also decreased. *Helps to increase blood flow to other, more active, tissues. Decreased motility reduces the demands made on tract muscle cells.*
Liver and adipose tissue	Metabolic fuels (glucose and fatty acids) are mobilized. *Meets the needs of increased metabolic activity in tissues such as skeletal muscle.*

hormone are highlighted in Table 7.2; these actions are discussed in detail in a later section (pp. 227–32). It is sufficient to note here that these actions mobilize the body's energy reserves.

■ An 'exhaustion' phase. According to Selye, failure to cope with the stressors will precipitate further alarm/resistance responses and eventually lead to exhaustion when physiological responses are no longer adequate or appropriate. This would be considered maladaptive, and carries potential risks for health.

The alarm and resistance phases facilitate our ability to cope with stressors. In other words, although it may seem that hormonal homeostasis in these phases has failed, the responses are examples of homeostatic adaptation (see Figure 7.2, and also Chapter 1).

Surgery as a stressor

The responses of the 'General Adaptation Syndrome' are adaptive in situations of psychological trauma, because they raise metabolic rate and, through the actions of adrenaline (epinephrine), heighten mental awareness and speed up reflexes. Whilst undoubtedly of importance here, the responses appear even more relevant

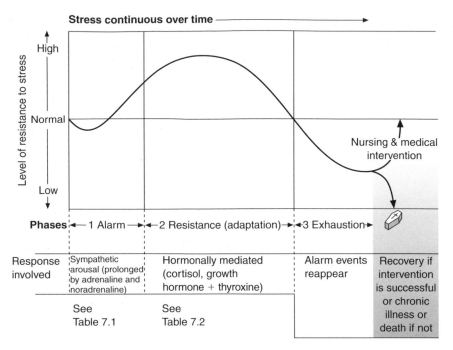

Figure 7.2 **Stress responses as a 'general adaptation syndrome'**
(See text, p. 214). The diagram follows the pattern suggested by Selye (1956) in which stress responses are identified as promoting an alarm phase, resistance phase and exhaustion phase. Neural and/or hormonal mechanisms are identified for the phases. The graph forming the upper part of the figure identifies the phases in relation to homeostatic adaptation

Q. How do stress responses relate to homeostatic theory? You might find it helpful to refer to Chapter 1 in considering this.

to a much more basic threat to an individual's existence: physical trauma. Surgical procedures cause such trauma and the role of responses in promoting homeostasis are explored later.

Surgical stress influences homeostasis in three ways.

1   Through the impact of anxiety that is generated by the perioperative situation. The anxiety that is understandably produced when an individual is faced with surgery is an obvious expression of stress, and is an example of 'mind–body' interaction operating via the autonomic nervous system. On the whole, this is a negative influence and so is maladaptive.

2   Through the potentially depressive effects of anaesthesia. Although anaesthesia cannot be considered a conventional stressor, general anaesthetics do have inhibitory actions on the brain stem, where much of sympathetic nerve activity originates, having potential consequences for body functioning that

Table 7.2 Main actions of cortisol, growth hormone and thyroxine
Consequences of the actions are highlighted in *italics* and are discussed in the text (pp. 227–32). A summary is provided that highlights the hormonal contribution to wound healing

	Cortisol	Growth hormone	Thyroxine
Effect on carbohydrate metabolism	Promotes glucose mobilization via gluconeogenesis (*increases blood glucose concentration*).	Promotes glucose mobilization via glycogenolysis but induces resistance to glucose uptake by cells and so promotes increase in blood glucose concentration (= '*diabetogenic*' *action; increases blood glucose concentration*).	Actions to promote basal respiration will increase utilization of glucose (*acts to increase basal metabolic rate*).
Effect on protein metabolism	Protein breakdown (proteolysis) in skeletal muscle (*increases availability of amino acids*).	Stimulates uptake of amino acids by cells and promotes protein synthesis (*promotes tissue growth*).	Actions to promote basal respiration will include utilization of amino acids (*acts to increase basal metabolic rate*).
Effect on lipid metabolism	Promotes fat breakdown (lipolysis) leading to releases of fatty acids (*increases blood concentration of free fatty acids, and their utilization by cells*).	Promotes fat catabolism leading to release of free fatty acids (*increases free fatty acid concentration in blood and their utilization by cells*).	Actions to promote basal respiration will include utilization of fatty acids (*acts to increase basal metabolic rate*).
Effect on immunity	Inhibits inflammatory responses. Inhibits development of fibroblasts and the process of fibrosis (*reduces scarring*).	No effect on immunity.	No effect on immunity.
Permissive effects	Exerts 'permissive' effects to increase the actions of other hormones (*potentiates cardiovascular actions of catecholamines*).	No 'permissive' effect on actions of other hormones.	Exerts 'permissive' effects to increase the actions of growth hormone and catecholamines (*potentiates the actions of growth hormone on tissue growth, and the cardiovascular actions of catecholamines*).
Summary	1. Elevates concentrations of metabolic fuels in blood. 2. Elevates concentration of amino acids in blood. 3. Contributes to wound healing. 4. Potentiates other hormones involved in the stress response.	1. Elevates concentrations of metabolic fuels in blood. 2. Promotes protein synthesis by cells, facilitating wound healing.	**1. Promotes utilization of metabolic fuels, and so provides more energy for wound healing.** **2. Potentiates other hormones involved in the stress response.**

are additional to the induction of a loss of consciousness, and so should be considered stressful. The consequences do not facilitate homeostasis and so are maladaptive.

3 Through the trauma induced by the surgical procedure itself. As noted above, in this context stress responses are beneficial and so are adaptive, although the persistence of metabolic changes can eventually lead to maladaptation.

These three aspects provide the structure of this chapter.

EXERCISE

Consider how you feel when you are stressed. Would you say that your response to the stress is adaptive or maladaptive?

Surgical stress I: anxiety

For many patients, admission to hospital for an operation heightens anxiety and so is very stressful (Welsh 2000). Furthermore, pre-operative anxiety may impact on the post-operative period, causing stress, pain and elevated anxiety levels. Reducing pre-operative anxiety therefore can have significant post-operative benefits. In particular there appears to be a positive impact on patient well-being, reduction of anxiety and compliance with treatment (Shuldham 1999). The evidence for positive outcomes for post-operative pain management and length of stay is more equivocal (Shuldham 1999) but the implication of research is that the patient experience is improved if pre-operative education is provided (Webb 1995; Shuldham 1999; Welsh 2000).

Anxiety produces symptoms of tachycardia, hyperventilation, sweating and agitation; all are indicative of sympathetic nerve activity (and adrenaline) and, according to Selye's General Adaptation Syndrome, conform to the alarm phase of the stress response (Figure 7.2; Table 7.1). Pre-operative sympathetic activity associated with anxiety could impact on the progress of surgery, especially in view of the cardiovascular and respiratory depressive effects of general anaesthetics. Anxiety may also exacerbate any underlying pathology, for example cardiac dysrhythmias may be exaggerated.

Fainting is another potential outcome of severe pre-operative anxiety. Fainting occurs if blood pressure falls below that necessary to maintain adequate blood supply to the brain. Although stress responses are usually associated with sympathetic nerve stimulation, fainting arising from anxiety is likely to be the result of a parasympathetic 'vasovagal' response; that is, activity in the vagus nerve from the brain stem to the heart induces a profound bradycardia and hence lowers arterial blood pressure. The response is exacerbated by a reduction in (accelerator) sympathetic activity to the heart via the cardiac nerves. Even in the absence of fainting, the sacral nerves of the parasympathetic division may act to increase muscle tension in the urinary bladder, conveying a feeling of urgency to pass urine.

Parasympathetic nerve activation is not part of the General Adaptation Syndrome but is clearly a stress response. The syndrome attempts to explain medium to long-term adaptation to stress, and the extreme effects of parasympathetic activation do not fit comfortably with this notion of adaptation. Fainting should be viewed as being an extreme response and one suggestion for its value is that it is a device which could be 'useful' when an individual's perception is that the threat will in all likelihood result in their death! This is a debatable viewpoint, but one which perhaps provides the rationale for reassuring the patient of the skills of the surgical team!

EXERCISE

Using an anatomy text, identify the organization of the sympathetic and parasympathetic branches of the nervous system.

Surgical stress II: general anaesthesia

Anaesthesia and the brain stem

Box 7.1   Application: pharmacology of general anaesthesia (see also Box 6.5)

What follows considers some aspects of the pharmacology of anaesthesia. Before continuing, readers might find it useful to review the actions and roles of excitatory and inhibitory synapses (see Box 2.7, and also the actions of pain 'gates' described in Chapter 8), and to define the terms 'non-depolarizing' and 'depolarizing' that are used in relation to the way muscle relaxants influence the generation of nerve impulses.

General anaesthesia consists of three phases: (a) loss of consciousness (or 'induction'), (b) pain relief and (c) muscle relaxation (Griffiths 2000). Each part has a different effect on neurological homeostasis of the whole body. The level of loss of consciousness, pain relief and muscle relaxation varies depending to the surgical procedure being performed and the physical condition of the patient.

Induction of anaesthesia

The first phase of a general anaesthetic is known as induction, and this can be achieved through intravenous injection or by inhalational anaesthetic agents. Two of the commonly used intravenous induction agents are propofol and thiopentone. Unconsciousness occurs within seconds. Inhalational anaesthetics, e.g. halothane, enflurane and isoflurane, are absorbed by diffusion across the alveolar–capillary membrane and so the uptake of inhalational agents takes longer than intravenous agents. Both types of induction agents can be used to maintain anaesthesia during surgery.

The actions of excitatory neurotransmitters, including those within the brain and in muscle synapses, are depressed by anaesthetic agents. Each type of tissue varies in its sensitivity to these agents. The mid-brain, which is especially responsible for consciousness, is one of the most sensitive of the excitable tissues. It is therefore possible to produce unconsciousness using small concentrations of anaesthetic agents, without profoundly depressing cardiac and respiratory function through actions on other brain stem nuclei, though such depressive actions remain a potential risk (Neal 1997; Griffith 2000).

Pain relief

The effect of the analgesic part of the 'anaesthetic' is difficult to assess once the patient is unconscious, partly because each drug produces a differing analgesic effect and there is varying sensitivity of the body tissues to these drugs. Additional opioid analgesics might be administered. The most commonly used opioid analgesics are fentanyl and morphine, which act on the pain synapses (see Figure 8.4; Chapter 8) within the spinal cord and mid-brain. Opioid analgesic drugs mimic the naturally occurring opioid peptides and cause prolonged activation of the opioid receptors, and 'close' the pain 'gates' (see Figure 8.6; Chapter 8).

Muscle relaxation

Neuromuscular blocking drugs act on the neuromuscular junction (a form of synapse) by competing with the transmitter chemical, acetylcholine, for its receptor. There are two main types of neuromuscular blocking agents, non-depolarizing and depolarizing. Non-depolarizing drugs act on the acetylcholine receptors to reduce the size of the ion channels in the muscle cell membrane, preventing the generation of muscle action potentials. Depolarizing drugs act on the acetylcholine receptors and trigger the opening of the ion channels causing brief muscle action potentials and muscle fibre twitching (fasciculation), followed by neuromuscular blockade.

Neuromuscular blocking drugs are administered by intravenous injection and are distributed in the extracellular fluid, therefore they do not cross the blood–brain barrier or the placenta and so do not influence cholinergic synapses within the brain or in the fetus. The choice of drug is largely dependent upon its side effects; some, for example pancuronium, produce tachycardia, whilst vecuronium and atracurium have no cardiovascular effects.

The duration of action for each of the muscle relaxants is dependent on the way in which they are excreted from the body. Atracurium is decomposed spontaneously in plasma (referred to as 'Hoffman degradation') and is useful in patients who have renal or hepatic disease, since the rate of renal or hepatic clearance of the drug will be reduced in these disorders; this duration of drug action is usually fifteen to thirty minutes. Vecuronium is dependent on hepatic inactivation and renal excretion, and recovery usually occurs within twenty to thirty minutes.

Suxamethonium is a depolarizing neuromuscular blocking drug. It is quickly broken down by plasma pseudo-cholinesterase (cholinesterase is an enzyme that removes acetylcholine from synaptic receptors); it has a rapid effect with a short duration of about three to seven minutes. However, in some people the effect can last for hours, due to an inherited atypical form of the enzyme, potentially producing apnoea that requires post-operative ventilation. The drug also causes twitching, which can result in muscle pain post-operatively (Neal 1997).

Today there are a number of ways in which anaesthesia is used to provide optimal conditions for surgical intervention. General anaesthesia, regional anaesthesia and regional analgesia are all methods of producing pain relief, and/or loss of consciousness, and/or muscle relaxation. The variety of surgical procedures and patient requirements dictate the type of anaesthesia and/or analgesia given (Carrie *et al.* 1997). General anaesthetics act on the brain stem to induce a loss of consciousness either by causing inhibition of excitatory nerve pathways, or by activating inhibitory nerve pathways: the precise mode of action is largely unknown. Regional anaesthesia and regional analgesia also have an effect on neurological homeostasis, but usually at a more local level (Chapter 8).

The brain stem is comprised of the mid-brain and parts of the hind-brain (the pons varolii and medulla oblongata; Figure 7.3). These structures contain:

- aggregates of nerve cell bodies, referred to as nuclei, that are integrating areas which help to co-ordinate various aspects of neurological functioning. Numerous nuclei are present (Figure 7.3) including the reticular formation (plus associated nuclei that together comprise the 'reticular-activating system'), respiratory centres and cardiovascular centres.
- (afferent) nerve pathways into and (efferent) pathways out of the fore-brain and cerebellum. Prominent efferent pathways are those referred to as the pyramidal tracts (the pyramids are large tracts of nerve fibres in the posterior surface of the brain stem) which carry neural activity from the motor areas of the cerebral cortex to the skeletal muscles.

EXERCISE

Readers unfamiliar with general brain anatomy are recommended to review the following terms: fore-brain, mid-brain, hind-brain, cerebral cortex and pyramidal tracts.

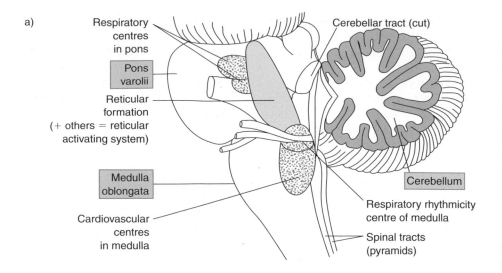

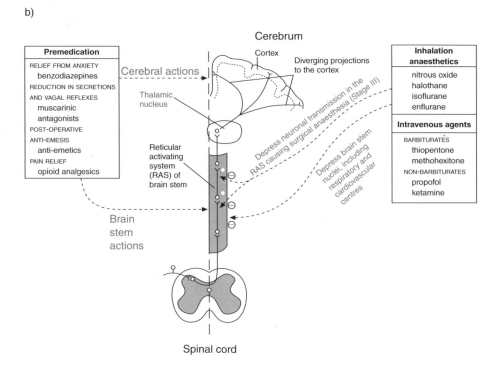

Figure 7.3 **The brain stem and actions of general anaesthetics**
a Brain stem; lateral view
b Actions of general anaesthetics.

Q. What is the role of the reticular activating system in: *a* **waking us up?** *b* **causing us to fall asleep?**

The reticular-activating system arouses the brain from sleep, and keeps it aroused whilst we are awake. It does this by sending impulses throughout the brain, especially to the cerebral cortex. 'Consciousness', however, implies something beyond arousal; a capacity of the brain to make us 'aware'. From a sensory viewpoint, consciousness means that we can consciously perceive our environment and interpret it in a meaningful way, though how this interpretation of sensory information occurs continues to elude science. Arousal of the cerebral cortex is essential to the process; by inhibiting the reticular-activating system, general anaesthetics diminish arousal and so reduce consciousness.

Box 7.2   Application: depressant actions of general anaesthetics

Direct effects of anaesthetic agents on tissues other than the brain stem were noted in Box 7.1. Significant effects may also arise if the anaesthetics also promote inhibition of additional parts of the brain stem, hence depressing their activities.

■ Depression of the cardiovascular centres lowers cardiovascular functioning, leading to bradycardia and hypotension. Hypotension stimulates blood pressure-restoring processes, most notably a release of vasoactive hormones (e.g. adrenaline, angiotensin II and vasopressin i.e. ADH), and stimulates sympathetic nerve activity. The consequence is vasoconstriction in various tissues (e.g. skin, gastrointestinal tract, kidneys) and hence a depression of their activities. Thus, kidney function may be compromised, and bowel stasis may be observed.

■ Depression of the respiratory centres may cause hypoventilation, therefore hypoxaemia and carbon dioxide retention. The latter will result in respiratory acidosis (see Chapter 6) and this may exacerbate any bradycardia caused by the anaesthetics (see above) and may even promote arrhythmias.

■ Deep anaesthesia causes depression of the pyramidal tracts leading to muscle relaxation. This action might actually be of benefit to the surgeon but the need for deep anaesthesia might have adverse consequences. Fortunately, the introduction of muscle relaxant drugs has removed the necessity for such deep anaesthesia, although this in itself may introduce problems with the patient's level of unconsciousness (Oulette and Oulette 1998).

Patient monitoring in the immediate post-operative period

The recovery room is a specialist area, which is fully equipped to provide close observation and monitoring of patients during this critical phase until they are able to return to the ward (Dennison 1997). The depressant effects of anaesthetic agents (Box 7.2) may extend into the post-operative period. In the absence of complications, regular observations of vital signs must be made during this period when much of the restoration of homeostasis takes place. As the patient recovers conciousness close clinical observation is essential, as early detection of problems and rapid intervention is paramount.

A scoring system may be used to assess the patient's stage of recovery. Respiration, circulation, level of consciousness and power, tissue perfusion, temperature, and the presence of pain and nausea are some of the essential observations that may be included in some scoring systems. An appropriate score will provide an indication that the patient may be fit for discharge from the recovery room (see Hatfield and Tronson 2000); however, a clinical assessment by the perioperative practitioner must also be considered prior to discharge.

Airway

Patency of the patient's airway must be ensured at all times, especially with the unconcious patient. If the patient is on their back, chin lift (head tilt) and jaw thrust (Chapter 6) may be required to prevent airway obstruction, or if the patient can be placed on their (left) side this will prevent the tongue from falling back and obstructing the airway. The airway may also become obstructed with vomit, blood or other secretions, and suction may be required to clear the airway. An oral or nasopharangeal airway may be used for airway maintainance, although some patients may require reintubation if the airway remains obstructed, for example in cases of laryngeal spasm.

Breathing

Alteration in the breathing movements can be an indication that the residual effects of anaesthesia may be affecting the patient's breathing. Antagonist drug therapy will reverse the effects of the anaesthetic drugs and stimulate the respiratory centre of the brain. It is common for patients to be given oxygen therapy during the recovery phase to aid breathing, help to eliminate vapour anaesthetics and reduce the risk of hypoxaemia (Chapter 6).

Circulation

Monitoring of the pulse, arterial blood pressure and electrocardiogram (ECG) is necessary to assess the patient's cardiovascular status. Any significant alteration may be an indication of cardiac, respiratory or neurological deficits which may be pre-existent or due to the anaesthetic drugs. Surgical problems, e.g. haemorrhage, will also alter the cardiovascular status (Chapter 5).

Level of conciousness

It is important to assess the level of conciousness as this provides evidence of reversal from anaesthesia and return of protective airway reflexes. For example, level of consciousness may be scored using four stages:

Stage 1: Patient unresponsive to shaking by the shoulder.
Stage 2: Patient is responsive to painful stimuli.
Stage 3: Patient is responsive to verbal stimuli.
Stage 4: Patient is awake and communicating.

Assessment of the response for its appropriateness will provide further evidence of the level of conciousness. A fully concious patient should be awake and responding appropriately to commands, although the influences of other drugs, e.g. analgesics, may cause drowsiness.

Fluid balance

Fluid input must be strictly measured according to the instructions of the medical staff. All fluid output should be accurately recorded, as should wound site exudate and haemorrhage, contents of drains, naso gastric tube drainage, urine, vomit and faeces. Any excess loss must be reported to the surgeon and/or anaesthetist concerned. Maintenance of fluid balance is essential to avoid overloading or dehydrating the patient (Chapter 3).

Pharmacology

The recovery time from drug actions can vary considerably:

- between individual patients,
- because of the type of surgery,
- because of the anaesthetic time,
- because of the type of anaesthetic given,
- because pain relief is used, and
- through any pre-existing clinical conditions which the patient may have.

Reversal or antagonist agents to reverse the effects of muscle relaxants, opioid analgesia or benzodiazepines may be necessary. Antibiotic, analgesic, diuretic, antihypertensive, antiemetic and resuscitation drugs are just a few of the drugs which might be required in the recovery phase (see Chapters 3, 4, 5, 6).

EXERCISE

The early post-operative period is a critical time for all patients. Many complications can occur and so individualized patient care is essential. Familiarize yourself with the specialist equipment that is required within the recovery area, and explore the role of the perioperative practitioner:

- when the cardiovascular status is compromised,
- when respiratory status is compromised,
- when the patient is unresponsive to pain or verbal stimulation.

Surgical stress III: responses to trauma

It was noted in the Introduction how the activation of sympathetic nerves, and the secretion of metabolic hormones, support the individual during and following physical injury. This section considers these aspects in more detail, and therefore discusses:

- the role of stress responses in supporting the cardiovascular system,
- the role of stress responses in promoting metabolism.

Supporting the cardiovascular system

The principles of cardiovascular homeostasis, and circulatory responses to surgery, are described in more detail in Chapter 5, and readers are recommended to re-visit this chapter. However, the cardiovascular actions of sympathetic nerves, supported by catecholamine hormones, represent an important part of the stress response to surgery and are worth reviewing here since they reinforce how stress responses facilitate homeostasis during and after trauma.

A significant loss of blood during surgery should be expected to stimulate sympathetic nerve activity, and to promote the release of vasoactive hormones (especially adrenaline, vasopressin and angiotensin II), which will promote cardiac function and increase peripheral resistance, the two determinants in blood pressure homeostasis. However, there is an additional aspect. Contact with, and manipulation of, internal organs is a very powerful stimulus for the release of these hormones regardless of blood loss (Shirasaka *et al.* 1986; Friedrich *et al.* 1999). In a 'natural' sense such contact would represent a severe trauma that would ordinarily be expected to induce haemorrhage and so the alarm response may also be viewed as being anticipatory of hypovolaemia. This helps to explain why abdominal and thoracic surgery, indicative of serious trauma, provide particularly powerful stimuli for the secretion of vasoactive hormones.

Surgery is a controlled trauma in that blood loss is minimized. With limited blood loss a powerful release of vasoactive hormones might be expected to elevate arterial blood pressure, but their actions are offset against the effects of anaesthetics, some of which may depress the brain stem control of the cardiovascular system (see earlier discussion, p. 223). Thus, the release of vasoactive hormones, and the influence of sympathetic nerve activity to blood vessels, will actually help to control arterial blood pressure in the presence of depressant effects of anaesthesia. The permissive actions of cortisol upon the actions of catecholamines provides additional support following trauma.

Further actions of adrenaline, vasopressin and angiotensin II include the promotion of blood clotting (adrenaline) and the initiation of water and electrolyte conservation (all three hormones, but especially vasopressin and angiotensin). These actions again are of obvious benefit should blood loss have occurred, but they will also have implications for the patient's water balance in the post-operative period (Chapter 3).

EXERCISE

Why is adrenaline usually associated with the sympathetic nervous system?

Metabolic responses to surgical stress

Strictly speaking, the term 'metabolism' covers all of the chemical processes that occur within the body. However, the term is usually equated with the production of the energy required to maintain those reactions. Indeed, the conventional method of determining an individual's metabolic rate is to calculate oxygen consumption, since aerobic respiration is the main route for energy production by cells. The complexity of the biochemical processes involved in respiration is apparent by taking just a cursory look at a biochemistry textbook, but understanding these principles is essential if the metabolic responses to surgery are to be appreciated. Accordingly, the first part of this section considers some aspects of metabolism in health, before going on to explore the implications of surgery.

EXERCISE

This section includes some difficult material. Readers may find it useful to consult a physiology textbook and clarify the process of 'respiration'; i.e. the production of energy by cells.

What do the terms 'aerobic respiration' and 'anaerobic respiration' mean?

Metabolic homeostasis in health

Carbohydrates, lipids and proteins comprise the main metabolic fuels and these therefore figure prominently in the average diet. To be precise, it is the simple sugars (ingested on their own or as components of larger, complex chemicals such as starch), fatty acids (components of lipid, especially fats) and amino acids (components of proteins) that form the actual fuels, and also provide the 'building blocks' of complex structural chemicals within cells.

These 'simple' substances are made available to tissues through the digestion of dietary constituents, and by their release from body stores. Some of the substances are interchangeable: for example, the simple sugar fructose can be converted in the liver to glucose, some amino acids can be converted to others or to glucose, and glycerol (another component of fats) can be converted to glucose. Such conversions highlight the flexibility of many metabolic processes but also emphasize the importance of glucose availability: recommendations are that on average about 55 per cent of the energy required by cell processes in health should be derived from the breakdown of glucose, the remainder from fatty acids (35 per cent) and amino acids (10 per cent) (Department of Health 1991).

Glucose enters cells by facilitated diffusion and so an adequate concentration gradient must exist between the extracellular and intracellular fluids. The concentration of glucose in blood plasma is therefore closely controlled in health; pronounced and persistent elevations in blood glucose concentration (= hyperglycaemia) must be avoided, as evidenced by the long-term health risks associated with uncontrolled diabetes mellitus, whilst a blood glucose concentration that is too low (=hypoglycaemia) will result in cells being starved of glucose and hence of energy.

Blood glucose concentration is determined by the balance between the rate of glucose utilization from blood and the addition of glucose to it. On a day-to-day basis, it is largely under the control of three pancreatic hormones: insulin, glucagon and somatostatin (Figure 7.4). The latter has a local role to modulate the actions of insulin and glucagon and so prevent any excessive responses to them. The actions of the others are discussed here.

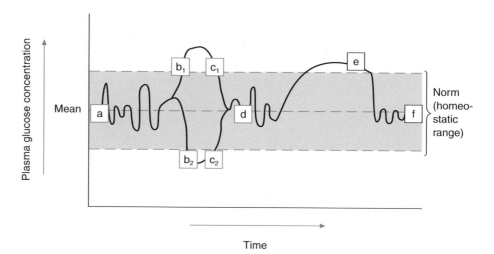

Figure 7.4 Blood glucose homeostasis
Blood glucose concentration is represented as a value that fluctuates but is maintained within a range which is appropriate for optimal function
a   Normal blood glucose concentration. Values fluctuating within the homeostatic range.
b_1 Glucose concentration increasing outside the homeostatic range (hyperglycaemia) after a meal.
b_2 Glucose concentration decreasing outside the homeostatic range (hypoglycaemia) as a consequence of fasting.
c_1 Reversal of hyperglycaemia via negative feedback. Process is mediated by insulin which increases glucose utilization or storage (see text, p. 229).
c_2 Reversal of hypoglycaemia via negative feedback. Normally mediated by glucagon.
d   Blood glucose homeostasis re-established.
e   During the perioperative period actions of adrenaline, cortisol and growth hormone alter the homeostatic balance with the consequence that glucose may exceed its normal plasma concentration and a hyperglycaemia persists.
f   As stress-hormone release declines to normal baseline values following surgery, blood glucose concentration returns to the normal homeostatic range.

Q. Why is the change c_2 referred to as a negative feedback?

Insulin

Insulin release is stimulated when blood glucose concentration increases following the absorption of carbohydrates from a digested a meal. The hormone promotes uptake of glucose into various insulin-sensitive tissues including the liver, skeletal muscle and fat cells. Glucose taken into cells may be utilized in three ways (Figure 7.5), although few tissues are capable of producing all three processes:

■   direct usage in energy production, or
■   conversion to storage carbohydrate (namely glycogen in liver and skeletal muscle, via the process of glycogenesis), or
■   conversion to non-carbohydrate substances such as glycerol and certain amino acids (which may be utilized in fat and protein synthesis respectively).

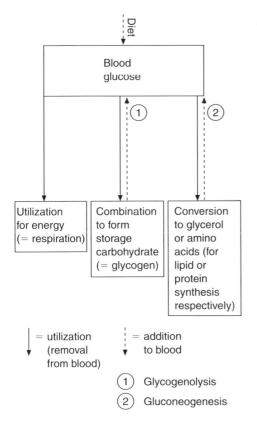

Figure 7.5 **Overview of glucose utilization. Note the reversibility of some processes**

Q. Where in the body would most of the conversions shown take place?

Glucagon

The utilization of glucose by cells means that the blood glucose concentration will begin to decrease between meals. Maintaining an adequate glucose concentration is therefore likely to necessitate the eventual release of glucose from storage (Figure 7.5) via:

- the breakdown of glycogen (a process referred to as glycogenolysis). Glycogen reserves of the body are very limited and account for only a proportion of the average daily energy requirement of an individual.
- the synthesis of glucose from non-carbohydrates (referred to as gluconeogenesis). As glycogen stores become depleted, the process of maintaining blood glucose concentration increasingly depends upon this process. Fat stores provide the main energy resource sources of substrate for gluconeogenesis; protein breakdown normally only serves as a reserve of energy if fat stores become depleted. Most fats within the body consist of glycerol combined with fatty acids and it is the glycerol that is used for glucose synthesis. The mobilization of fatty acids that occurs also represents an important additional energy source since these can also enter cells either directly, or as ketone bodies (acetoacetate, beta-hydroxybutyrate) produced from them by the liver, and provide a further source of energy.

EXERCISE

Imagine having just eaten a meal. What do you think happens to the release of the hormones insulin and glucagon in the period after eating, and during the period until you eat again?

Metabolic responses to surgery

Increased energy demands during wound healing require a resetting of glucose homeostatic set-points (Figure 7.4). Additional mobilization of glucose is promoted, leading to an elevation of blood glucose concentration. This is beneficial because it increases the concentration gradient to promote glucose influx into tissues, including into those such as the heart and brain which are not dependent upon the presence of insulin for glucose uptake. Glucose mobilization is achieved through the activity of the sympathetic nervous system, and the hormones adrenaline and cortisol, which stimulate glycogenolysis and gluconeogenesis. An elevation of blood glucose concentration is also facilitated by the action of growth hormone to promote resistance to insulin in insulin-dependent cells; these cells (e.g. skeletal muscle) comprise much of the body tissues and this insulin resistance will make them more dependent upon fatty acids for energy. The availability of these fuels is not a problem, however, since break-down of fat for gluconeogenesis also liberates fatty acids.

> **Box 7.3   Application: metabolic phases in recovery from surgery**
>
> Surgical trauma promotes metabolic responses that can be divided into various phases. In particular:
>
> - following surgery the individual rapidly enters a phase in which there is reduced metabolic rate but the concentration of metabolic fuels within the blood increases. This phase is usually quite short and might actually start prior to injury due to responses associated with the 'alarm' phase of stress responses, as identified by Selye (1956), as adrenaline promotes gluconeogenesis.
> - after several hours the individual enters a phase characterized by an increased metabolic rate: these responses may be substantial, especially after severe trauma.
>
> In this context metabolism is considered to 'ebb and flow', and the second phase is frequently referred to as the 'flow phase'. Although longer-term phases can also be identified during which the metabolic status of the individual returns to normal, it is the flow phase that covers the immediate week or so after surgery, and so it is within this period that the major adaptive responses for recovery are observed.

Despite these changes, basal metabolism does not actually increase overall during the 'ebb' phase (see Box 7.3 for an explanation of metabolic phases in surgery), and often decreases, suggesting that there are additional biochemical adaptations. However, the 'ebb' phase is usually quite short and the individual soon enters the 'flow' phase when these metabolic responses facilitate an increased metabolic rate.

EXERCISE

At this point it would be useful to remind yourself what 'basal metabolic rate' means, what its significance is to clinical practice, and to identify the factors which might influence it during the post-operative period.

Gluconeogenesis from amino acids entails protein breakdown in order to release the amino acids required (Molina *et al.* 1998). This also results in an increased production and urinary excretion of urea (a 'waste' product of amino acid breakdown), and of 3-methylhistidine: the presence of the latter in urine is indicative of muscle protein loss. Muscle provides the main source of protein in the body, but increased protein breakdown may also decrease the concentration of some plasma proteins, although fibrinogen (an important clotting protein) and antibodies may increase perhaps as haemostatic and anti-infection mechanisms, respectively.

The flow phase responses are summarized in Figure 7.6. The elevated metabolism observed during the flow phase causes:

■ body temperature to increase (this could be confused as indicating the presence of a mild infection),
■ an elevation in heart rate (to promote effective circulation), and
■ an elevation in lung ventilation (to promote oxygen uptake and carbon dioxide excretion).

The significance of increased mobilization of metabolic fuel is that it facilitates cell division, tissue growth and repair.

A further significance of the increased secretion of cortisol is that it eventually acts to reduce immune responses triggered by the injury, in particular inflammation. Although this might at first seem detrimental to recovery from surgery, the response is probably important later in the flow phase when the persistence of inflammation and fibrosis would act to hinder wound healing.

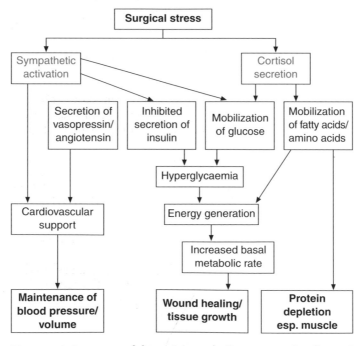

Figure 7.6 **Summary of the main metabolic events in the 'flow' phase of recovery from surgery**
Note how the net effect of the responses is generally one of facilitating recovery, apart from the metabolic 'cost' of protein depletion

Q. Refer to the text and identify why protein depletion might be a problem following surgery.

Surgery and diabetes mellitus

Diabetes mellitus is a condition characterized by a failure of the tissues to metabolize glucose adequately, and arises because there is inadequate production/ secretion of insulin, or inadequate responses to it. If uncontrolled, hyperglycaemia will be present, and tissues will excessively utilize other metabolic fuels, namely fatty acids and amino acids (from fats and proteins respectively). One risk of utilizing these fuels is that the cells produce excessive amounts of ketoacids as side-products and these may promote a metabolic acidosis. Further details on metabolism are provided in Clancy and McVicar (2002, Chapter 4).

The person with diabetes is faced with additional hazards from the imposition of metabolic responses to surgery upon an already disturbed metabolism (Marshall 1996). Under these circumstances the responses described previously that are ordinarily adaptive can become maladaptive and so have immediate implications for health. In diabetes, the shortage of insulin, or the presence of insulin resistance, exacerbates the metabolic response to surgery. The risks associated with this are:

- enhanced hyperglycaemia with the associated risk of hyperosmolar coma. Polyuria and polydipsia would also be expected,
- increased fatty acid mobilization to the extent that the risk of ketoacidosis is increased.

Such risks mean that monitoring blood glucose concentration accurately, and having to pay particular attention to maintaining the patient's metabolic control, will be important aspects for perioperative care of people with diabetes mellitus.

EXERCISE

Review your understanding of the two main types of diabetes mellitus and consider how metabolic control might be achieved with each type after surgery. Reference to Marshall (1996) might help.

Box 7.4   Application: implications of stress responses for recovery from surgery

The metabolic responses to surgery described in the text represent a resetting of homeostatic parameters, and so promote the functional changes necessary for recovery. According to stress theory (Clancy and McVicar 2002, Chapter 22), they provide adaptive mechanisms that promote the return to health of the individual. However, there is a metabolic 'cost' of the flow phase. Thus, fat stores may be reduced and, more significantly, the breakdown of muscle proteins caused by growth hormone and cortisol during the flow phase induces a loss of muscle tissue (Molina *et al.* 1998). The resultant increase in urea production from amino acid metabolism promotes a negative nitrogen balance, since urea contains nitrogen from amino acid breakdown. A persistence of protein depletion may hinder long-term wound healing (Rollins 1997; Carlson 1999) and also has implications for the general welfare of patients.

Wound healing will be enhanced, and protein depletion reduced, by ensuring that the patient has adequate protein nutrition during the flow phase. A good-quality diet should be available to patients, although commercially available supplements may also be used (Rollins 1997) in order to minimize protein depletion.

> **EXERCISE**
>
> The mineral zinc, and the vitamins A, C and E are especially important in wound healing. The vitamins support cell growth and tissue integrity, but what of zinc? To answer this you might refer to Andrews and Gallagher-Allred (1999).

Summary

- The General Adaptation Syndrome put forward by Selye almost fifty years ago is accepted as a description of the physiological responses observed when the body is subject to stress.
- Stress induces changes that involve the sympathetic nervous system and various hormones and, superficially, would appear to represent a significant failure of the homeostatic process.
- Pre-operative anxiety is viewed negatively and evidence suggests that patient well-being in the post-operative period is improved if pre-operative anxiety is reduced.
- General anaesthetics act on the brain stem to induce a loss of consciousness. Depressant actions on cardiovascular and respiratory control centres of the brain stem are a potential associated risk, as are additional stressors during the perioperative period.
- Persistence of depressant effects into the post-operative period makes patient monitoring a vital activity.
- Stress responses to the physical trauma introduced by surgery help maintain the circulatory system and facilitate wound healing, and should be viewed as being of benefit to recovery from surgery.
- The pronounced metabolic responses to surgical trauma have identifiable advantages, but the extent of the changes promoted by those responses also serve to reinforce why a level of control is essential even in health.
- Metabolic responses to stress hormones are influenced by factors such as sensitivity and an altered metabolic baseline; under these circumstances optimal conditions may not prevail, or the adaptive responses may themselves

promote a metabolic 'deficit', and thus the responses could have consequences for general well-being and recovery.

■ Nutritional support and the use of fluid therapies are therefore important considerations in the post-operative care of the surgical patient, especially if there is a pre-existing metabolic disturbance such as diabetes mellitus. In the latter case, even normal adaptive responses can act as a distressor.

■ Chapter 1 identified that homeostasis is not about constancy or even balance, but it is about the provision of optimal conditions. In this context stress responses should not necessarily be viewed as negative, but as enabling adaptation to the disturbance produced by physical trauma. However, the mechanisms that operate are also activated by anxiety and by anaesthesia and in these contexts can be negative and maladaptive.

Bibliography

Andrews, M. and Gallagher-Allred, C. (1999) The role of zinc in wound healing. *Advances in Wound Care* 12(3): 137–8.

British National Formulary (2002) *British National Formulary* (41). London: BMA/Royal Pharmaceutical Society.

Carlson, G.L. (1999) The influence of nutrition and sepsis upon wound healing. *Journal of Wound Care* 8(9): 471–4.

Carrie, L.E.S., Simpson, P.J. and Popat, M.T. (1997) *Understanding Anaesthesia, Third Edition.* Oxford: Butterworth Heinemann.

Case, R.M. and Waterhouse, J.M. (1994) *Human Physiology: Age, Stress and the Environment.* Oxford: Oxford University Press.

Clancy, J. and McVicar, A.J. (2002) *Physiology and Anatomy: A Homeostatic Approach, Second Edition.* London: Arnold.

Dennison, R.D. (1997) Nurse's guide to common postoperative complications. *Nursing* 27(11): 56–9.

Department of Health (1991) *Dietary Reference Values for Food Energy and Nutrients for the UK.* London: HMSO.

Forrest, A.P.M., Carter, D.C. and Macleod, I.B. (1995) *Principles and Practice of Surgery, Third Edition.* London: Churchill Livingstone.

Friedrich, M., Rixecker, D. and Friedrich, G. (1999) Evaluation of stress-related hormones after surgery. *Clinical and Experimental Obstetrics and Gynecology* 26(2): 71–5.

Garbee, D.D. and Gentry, J.A. (2001) Coping with the stress of surgery. *AORN Journal* 73(5): 946–51.

Greenfield, S. (2000) *The Private Life of the Brain.* London: Penguin.

Griffiths, R. (2000) Anaesthetic drugs. *British Journal of Perioperative Nursing* 10(5): 276–9.

Hatfield, A. and Tronson, M. (2000) *The Complete Recovery Room Book, Second Edition.* Oxford: Oxford University Press.

Marshall, S.M. (1996) The perioperative management of diabetes. *Care of the Critically Ill* 12(2): 64–7.

Molina, P.E., Ajmal, M. and Abumrad, N.N. (1998) Energy metabolism and fuel mobilization: from the perioperative period to recovery. *Shock* 9(4): 241–8.

Morgan, V. (1995) Brain stem death testing and consent for cadaveric organ donation. *Care of the Critically Ill* 11(1): 20–2.

Neal, M.J. (1997) *Medical Pharmacology at a Glance, Third Edition.* Oxford: Blackwell Science.

Oulette, S.M. and Oulette, R.G. (1998) Monitoring for intraoperative awareness: what's new? *Current Reviews for Perianaesthesia Nurses* 20(10): 107–13.

Rollins, H. (1997) Nutrition and wound healing. *Nursing Standard* 21(51): 49–52.

Selye, H. (1956) The general adaptation syndrome and diseases of adaptation. *Journal of Clinical Endocrinology* 6: 117–18.

Shirasaka, C., Tsuji, H., Asoh, T. and Takeuchi, Y. (1986) Role of the splanchnic nerves in endocrine and metabolic response to abdominal surgery. *British Journal of Surgery* 73: 142–5.

Shuldham, C. (1999) A review of the impact of pre-operative education on recovery from surgery. *International Journal of Nursing Studies* 36: 171–7.

Webb, R.A. (1995) Preoperative visiting from the perspective of the theatre nurse. *British Journal of Nursing* 4(16): 919–25.

Welsh, J. (2000) Reducing patient stress in theatre. *British Journal of Perioperative Nursing* 10(6): 321–7.

Chapter 8

Pain and pain relief in the perioperative patient

Introduction

Perioperative practitioners are certain to encounter patients in pain during perioperative care. In acute situations the surgical patient is often admitted in pain and post-operative pain is a normal consequence of surgery itself. A considerable number of patients discharged from hospital are in pain. The problem of inadequate pain control may be enhanced further; as there are increasing numbers of patients undergoing day case or short-stay surgery (Dobson 1997). Thus, there is a need for better education of healthcare professionals about pain control. In support of the statement we believe that perioperative practitioners must have a sound knowledge of the neurophysiology associated with pain, since this would be helpful in the understanding of the site of action of analgesic methods and anaesthesia employed during the perioperative period.

The chapter begins with a definition of pain, followed by the neurophysiology associated with Melzack and Wall's gate control theory of pain perception. An integrated science perspective using the nature–nurture interactions as a template will be used to explain the gate control theory. This involves linking the sociopsychology with the neurophysiology associated with pain perception. Finally, the site of action of pharmacological and non-pharmacological agents employed by the healthcare professional to control pain will be mentioned, with particular focus on perioperative care.

Definition of pain

Most people think they know what pain is and yet, from a scientific point of view, much still has to be discovered. Torrance and Serginson (1997) acknowledge this; they state that pain is one of the most misunderstood problems in surgical nursing.

Because of its importance in medicine, nursing and allied healthcare professions, any credible definition must include the subjective nature of pain, as emphasized by McCaffery's (1983) famous definition that:

> Pain is whatever the experiencing person says it is, existing whenever he says it does.

Pain perception: an overview

Pain perception is a function of the sensory nervous system (Kittelberger and Borsook 1996). It basically involves five components (see Figure 8.1).

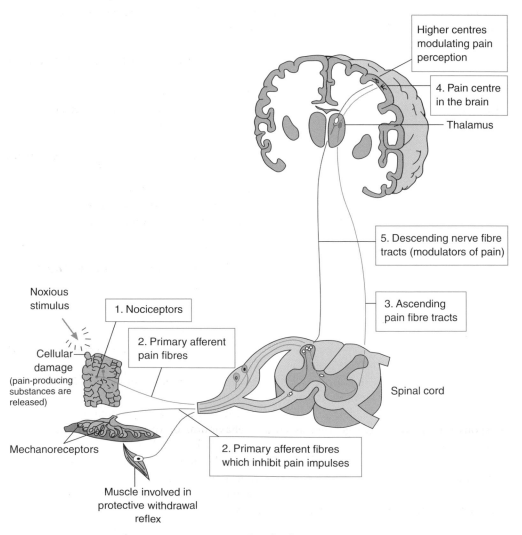

Figure 8.1 **The sensory components involved in pain perception**
See text, pp. 238–48, for details

1 Specialized pain receptors (nociceptors)

It is unclear what constitutes a pain receptor. Some nociceptors are probably free nerve endings, which are only sensitive to chemicals (e.g. bradykinin, lactic acid and prostaglandins) perhaps released from damaged cells in the vicinity. These are classified as a type of chemoreceptor. Other nociceptors are complex encapsulated structures sensitive to pronounced mechanical deformation (e.g. stretching, crushing, tearing, cutting) or extreme temperature change (e.g. scalding, burning and freezing). These are classified as types of mechanoreceptors and thermoreceptors respectively. Some nociceptors respond to only one type of stimulus, whilst others are capable of responding to all three (i.e. chemical, mechanical and thermal) stimuli and are known as polymodal nociceptors. Nociceptors are attached to distal ends of primary afferent pain fibres.

2 Primary afferent pain fibres

Primary pain afferents are sensory fibres that transmit the pain message as an electrical impulse from the receptors towards the central nervous system. Other primary afferents function to inhibit the passage of pain impulses.

3 Ascending nerve fibre tracts

The ascending pain fibre tracts are stimulated by a pain neurotransmitter released from the primary afferent pain fibres at synapses throughout the dorsal horn of grey matter spinal cord (and certain brain sites). They then conduct the pain impulse to the higher pain centres of the brain.

4 Higher pain centres of the brain

The higher pain centres interpret the electrochemical impulse conducted in pain fibres, originally derived from the noxious stimuli, as a perception of pain.

5 Descending nerve fibre tracts

The descending nerve fibre systems from the brain to the spinal cord are involved in modulating the perception of pain.

Once pain has been perceived, the body responds in a variety of ways. Responses to pain are categorized as either behavioural or those instigated by sympathetic activity. The former responses include vocal responses (e.g. moaning); verbal statements (e.g. 'ouch that hurts'); facial expression (e.g. grimacing); restricting movement and/or adopting a guarding behaviour ('protective rigidity'). Sympathetic responses include nausea, vomiting, gastric stasis, decreased gut motility and impaired renal activity.

Details of the neurophysiology associated with pain perception

Pain is generated usually in response to cellular damage. This may arise as a result of a surgical incision, traumatic injury, tumours compressing surrounding soft tissues, myocardial infarction, and so on. Tissue damage promotes the appearance of the classic signs of inflammation. A variety of chemicals accompany inflammation, secreted from nerve endings, blood vessel walls, phagocytes, lymphocytes and tissue cells as a number of homeostatic reflexes go into operation to promote the healing of the damaged tissue. These chemicals are responsible for promoting the familiar localized signs (i.e. swelling – oedema; redness – erythema; heat – vasodilation and pain) of the inflammatory process (see Chapter 4). This chapter is only concerned with those chemicals that induce pain, and those that enhance responses to painful stimuli.

Pain-producing substances

Pain-producing substances released from damaged tissue include histamine, kinin-like compounds such as bradykinin, and prostaglandins.

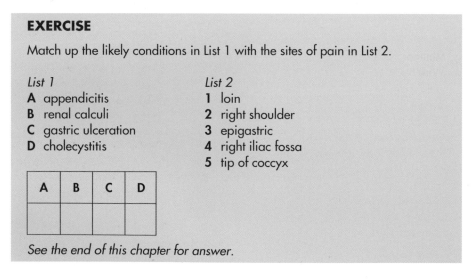

EXERCISE

Match up the likely conditions in List 1 with the sites of pain in List 2.

List 1
A appendicitis
B renal calculi
C gastric ulceration
D cholecystitis

List 2
1 loin
2 right shoulder
3 epigastric
4 right iliac fossa
5 tip of coccyx

A	B	C	D

See the end of this chapter for answer.

These substances combine with receptor binding sites on nociceptors – the initiators of the neural transmission associated with the perception of pain. In order to initiate a neural impulse, the interaction between pain-producing substances and nociceptors must reach the individual's pain threshold. The brain interprets the intensity of pain according to the number of pain impulses it receives within a set period of time. That is, the more impulses it receives, the greater the intensity of pain (see Figure 8.2). Their actions will now be considered in turn.

The secretion of histamine from basophils (also known as mast cells) is instigated by a number of chemical mediators including interleukin 1 and nerve growth factor, released in the vicinity of damaged tissue. At low concentration,

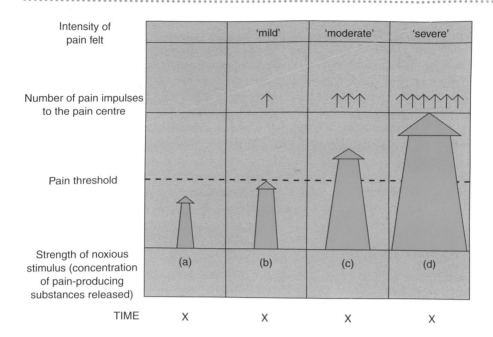

Figure 8.2 Pain threshold and the intensity of pain perception
a Minimal tissue damage, threshold not met, no pain impulse, no pain felt.
b More tissue damage, threshold reached, few pain impulses sent to the pain centre, 'mild' pain felt.
c Further tissue damage, threshold superseded, more pain impulses sent to the pain centre, 'moderate' pain felt.
d Severe tissue damage, threshold superseded further, many more pain impulses sent to the pain centre, 'severe' pain felt.

Q. Using the text and this figure distinguish between the following:
■ pain perception threshold,
■ severe pain threshold,
■ pain tolerance.

histamines stimulate sensory neurons to produce an itching sensation; at high concentrations these chemicals evoke a painful sensation.

Kinins sensitize polymodal nociceptors to heat and mechanical stimuli.

Prostaglandins are among the most important initiators of pain. These chemicals are synthesized from a modified fatty acid called arachidonic acid aided by the enzyme prostaglandin synthetase. Prostaglandins sensitize nociceptors, thereby enhancing the effects of other pain-producing substances and accordingly these chemicals may be considered the most important pain-producing substances in the human body (Clancy and McVicar 2002). They also enhance pain fibre response to non-noxious stimuli in polymodal nociceptors.

Nociceptors are located extensively in the dermal layer of the skin (Figure 2.1), periosteum (layer of fibrous tissue surrounding bones), articular surfaces of joints, walls of arteries and the dura mater (outer membrane covering the spinal cord and brain). Deeper tissues, particularly the walls of the viscera (internal organs), are less extensively supplied. Cutaneous pain receptors have a relatively high threshold. Thus a strong stimulus is required to generate an electrical signal which initiates the train of events resulting in pain perception.

EXERCISES

1 List the pain-producing substances released from cells following injury caused by, for example, a surgical incision.

2 Suggest why prostaglandins are considered by the authors and other theorists to be the most important pain-producing substances in the human body.

Anatomical location of nociceptors

Nociceptors are located at the distal end of afferent pain neurons. These neurons are small diameter, myelinated A-delta (δ) fibres and smaller unmyelinated C-fibres. These are classified as the 'fast' and 'slow' pain fibres respectively, since faster transmission is associated with thicker fibres and the presence of a myelin sheath. The A-δ fibres conduct messages at a speed of 5–25 metres per second; C-fibres conduct messages at 0.5–2 metres per second. Nociceptors for fast pain fibres are only located in the skin and mucous membranes, whilst nociceptors for slow pain fibres are found in the skin, and most other body tissues, except brain tissue which is insensitive to pain.

Box 8.1   Application: sharp and dull pains and reflexes – aids to diagnosing

If the perioperative pain is described by the patient as being sharp and prickling, this informs the practitioner that the pain fibres involved are mainly of the A-δ type. This type of pain can be precisely located by the patient because A-δ fibre nociceptors send pain signals along discrete pathways to the somatosensory cortex of the brain, which enables the pain to be established to within a few centimetres of the source (Woolf 1995).

EXERCISE

The reader is referred to a physiology textbook to identify the location of the somatosensory areas of the brain.

Fast pain is often simultaneously accompanied by withdrawal reflexes, activated via flexor motor neurons in the anterior horns of the spinal cord (Woolf 1995) that activate the effector organ, usually a muscle, to instigate a protective withdrawal contraction in an attempt to avoid any further damage (Figure 8.1). This reflex exhibits itself when one is cut with a sharp instrument such as a scalpel in the absence of an anaesthetic. To the trained practitioner protective withdrawal reflexes may be used to establish the origin of the damage, and thus may be considered an aid to diagnosis. For example, when a patient instinctively covers the right lower quadrant of the abdomen or left side of the chest, the practitioner may suspect the pain/damage is of appendix or cardiac origin respectively. This knowledge together with other signs and symptoms may aid a diagnosis of appendicitis and angina.

EXERCISE

See Figure 1.5 if you cannot visualize the location of the right lower quadrant of the abdomen.

If the assessment indicates that the pain is of a characteristically dull, burning, troublesome, aching, poorly localized and persistent nature, and is somatic in origin, it informs the practitioner that the pain fibres involved are of the C- variety (Kittleberger and Borsook 1996). Torrance and Serginson (1997) proposed that the immediate pain of a surgical incision is mediated by A-δ fibres, but within a few seconds the pain becomes more widespread due to C-fibre activation.

EXERCISE

Before going any further it is important to review from an anatomy and physiology textbook:

a the relative distribution of sodium and potassium ions on either side of the cell membrane of neurons required in establishing the resting membrane potential.

b the movement of these ions during the depolarized, repolarized and hyperpolarized phases of the action potential.

c Once you have reviewed a and b now revise the overview section in this chapter and reflect on your understanding of the components of the nervous system involved in the perception of pain.

The 'gate' control theory

Melzack and Wall in 1965 proposed a gating mechanism within the dorsal horn of grey matter of the spinal cord. These gates were the layer of cells called the substantia gelatinosa, through which sensory (afferent) pain impulses have to pass before they are relayed to, and perceived in, the 'pain centre' (or centres) of the brain. It is now generally accepted that every neuron is a 'gate'. The gates are symbolic of synapses between afferent neurons and various ascending and descending tract neurons. The gate control theory suggests that information can only pass through when the gate is 'open' and not when the gate is 'closed'. The opening of the gate is by the release at the synapse of excitatory neurotransmitter chemicals. The closing of the gate is brought about by the release of other chemicals, which are inhibitory neurotransmitters and neuromodulators (see Figure 8.3).

EXERCISE

Before continuing, review the relevant sections in a physiology textbook for a discussion on the involvement of excitatory and inhibitory neurotransmitters in synaptic conduction.

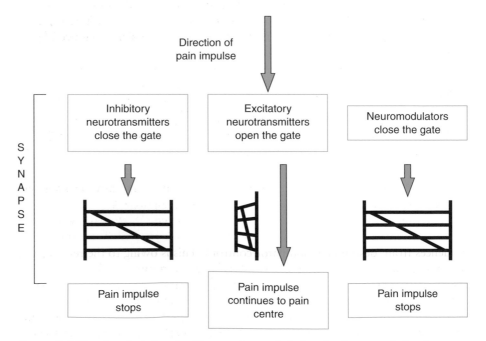

Figure 8.3 The chemicals involved in opening and closing the 'gateway' of pain

Q. Name the pain-producing substances mentioned in this chapter.

The reader is advised to look at Figures 8.3 and 8.4 whilst reading the following section since it will help your understanding of this complex topic.

The gating mechanism depends upon two modifying factors:

- the balance of activity of primary afferent (sensory) neurons,
- the modulator control of pain provided by descending fibres from the brain's higher centres.

Primary afferent fibre input

The afferent neurons, which provide input to the gate, are:

1   the nociceptors containing A-δ and C-pain fibres. These neurons release substance P, an excitatory neurotransmitter, at synapses (i.e. 'gates') within the central nervous system; and

2   the mechanoreceptors containing thick myelinated faster-transmitting A-beta (β) neurons. These fibres release inhibitory neurotransmitters (e.g. serotonin) at synapses within the central nervous system.

If the dominant input to the gate is via the faster-transmitting A-β fibres, then the gate will close due to the release and action of the inhibitory neurotransmitters.

Box 8.2   Application: reduce the pain associated with injection

Before giving an injection, some healthcare professionals and clinicians pinch the area to be injected to activate mechanoreceptors A-β fibre input to the pain gate, thereby reducing or inhibiting the pain signals induced by the penetrating needle.

EXERCISE

Using a physiology textbook review the conduction properties of myelinated A-δ and A-β fibres (i.e. saltatory transmission) and unmyelinated neurons C-pain fibres (i.e. local circuitry, non-saltatory transmission).

There are many potential sites of action of these inhibitory neurotransmitters (Clancy and McVicar 2002). These are summarized in Figure 8.4.

In contrast, if the dominant input to the gate is from the afferent A-Δ and/or C-pain fibres, the gate may be open (see later section, pp. 247–8, for additional influences from 'descending modulator control'). This is owing to the release, and the post-synaptic action, of the excitatory neurotransmitter substance P (see Figure 8.4). The pain impulse passes from the dorsal horn of grey matter in ascending pathways which, in the main, cross to the opposite side's (lateral) anterior commissure of the spinal cord before relaying upwards to the thalamus of the brain. These pathways are logically called the *anterolateral spinothalamic* ascending pain tracts. Some ascending pain fibre tracts (referred to as 'ipsilateral spinothalamic tracts', ips- = same) relay upwards to the thalamus whilst remaining on the same side of the cord.

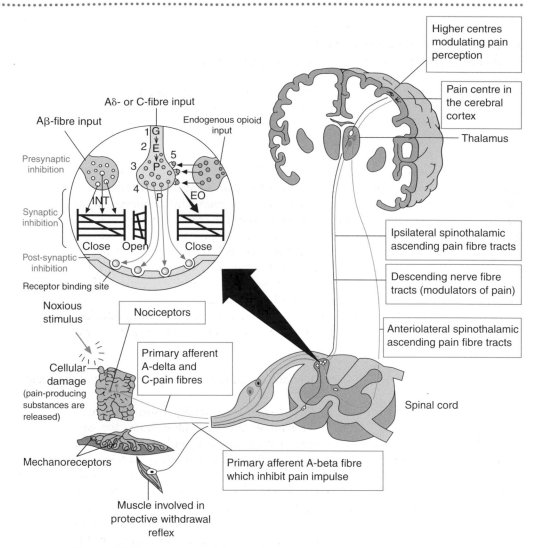

Figure 8.4 The gate control theory of pain perception
INT, Inhibitory neurotransmitters
EO, Endogenous opioids (neuromodulators)
P, Substance P

Q. Outline the principles behind the 'gate control theory' of pain perception, using the following terms: pain-producing substances; inhibitory neurotransmitters; excitatory neurotransmitters; neuromodulators; nociceptor; endogenous opioids; A-δ pain fibres; C-pain fibres; A-β fibres; threshold; afferent input; descending fibres; pain centre; higher cortical centres, kinins, prostaglandins, endorphins, enkephalins.

Q. Differentiate between the following:
a nociceptor and polymodal nociceptors.
b inhibitory neurotransmitters and excitatory neurotransmitters.

Q. Identify the possible sites of action of inhibitory neurotransmitters and Endogenous opioids. Use the text if you are experiencing difficulty.

The majority of A-δ fibres terminate in the thalamus, where they synapse with further neurons that transmit the signals to other basal areas of the brain and to the somatosensory cortex. Up to one quarter of the C-pain fibres terminate in the thalamus; the rest terminate in three distinct areas of the brain stem. Melzack and Wall (1996) state that the cerebral cortex may not contain specific pain centres, and it may just process the information it receives before transmitting it deeper into the brain tissue. It is generally believed that pain is felt in the mid-brain but the appreciation of its unpleasant qualities depends on the cerebral cortex. Thus, a specific pain centre (or centres) has not yet been located.

Pain perception will still only occur, however, if there is no or insufficient interference via descending fibre input to the gate from higher centres of the brain.

Descending modulator control from higher centres of the brain

The gate theory proposes that, even if pain A-δ and C- fibre input into the central nervous system dominates over the mechanoreceptor A-β fibre input, the gate may still be closed. This is because areas of the brain stem, such as the reticular formation, raphe nuclei, trigeminal nuclei, vestibular nuclei together with various nuclei of the hypothalamus and cerebral cortex, can modify the gating process via descending neural mechanisms. These are termed pain inhibitory complexes in the dorsal horns of the spinal cord (Stamford 1995). The neurons of this descending fibre system release a variety of endogenous opioids (enkephalins, endorphins and dynorphins). These neuromodulators bind to opioid receptor sites on the presynaptic membrane of the pain fibres and 'close the gate' by inhibiting the release of the pain neurotransmitter, substance P (see Figure 8.4). Because of their function these opioids have been referred to as the body's own natural 'pain killers' (Clancy and McVicar 2002). The distribution of opioid binding sites has been found to be uneven, with the highest concentration in the limbic system, thalamus, hypothalamus, mid-brain and spinal cord (Thomas 1996).

The reticular formation projects from the brain stem to exert a powerful inhibitory control over the spinal gating mechanism. These projections are also influenced via somatic (body) input, and input from auditory and visual centres. In addition, cortical projections, particularly from the frontal cortex (this area subserves cognitive processes, such as past experience) also pass to the reticular formation to mediate the control over the spinal gating mechanism. Cognitive processes can also influence gating mechanisms directly via their large fast conducting corticospinal (pyramidal) fibre tracts (see Figure 8.5). Melzack and Wall in 1965 proposed the idea of a 'central trigger' which activates particular brain processes, such as past experience and memories. Psychological processes play an extremely important role in pain perception, and research has shown those psychological factors such as anxiety and helplessness can intensify the pain experienced. Thus interventions that reduce anxiety or helplessness can reduce the pain experience and enhance coping (Thomas *et al.* 1995).

EXERCISE

Now it is time to test your understanding.

Using your own words in association with the statements and terms below, outline the principles underpinning Melzack and Wall's 'gate control theory' of pain perception.

Cellular damage resulting from a surgical incision; secretion of pain-producing substances; secretion of inhibitory neurotransmitters; secretion of excitatory neurotransmitters; perioperative practitioner employs her/his communicative skills to allay anxiety in her/his patients; neuromodulators; nociceptors; endogenous opioids; A-δ pain fibres; C-pain fibres; A-β fibres; threshold; afferent input; descending fibres; pain centre; higher cortical centres; kinins; prostaglandins; endorphins; enkephalins; substance P; decrease the patient's pain perception.

The following section now attempts to explain from a biochemical perspective why pain is considered to be a subjective phenomenon.

The subjectivity of pain

Pain is a subjective experience since each individual has a unique range of anatomical, physiological, social and psychological identities. These identities using the nature–nurture interactions template can be applied to the gate control theory to help to explain the subjective nature of pain perception. The concept of individualized pain relief is based upon this template application to the gate theory.

Anatomical subjectivity

The size and shape of the human body is genetically controlled and environmentally modified. Thus a tremendous variation in human body shapes and sizes exists and it is not surprising, therefore, that the distribution of nociceptors and hence pain fibres varies between individuals. This could be expected to produce regional variations of anatomical subjectivity, in sensitivity to stimuli.

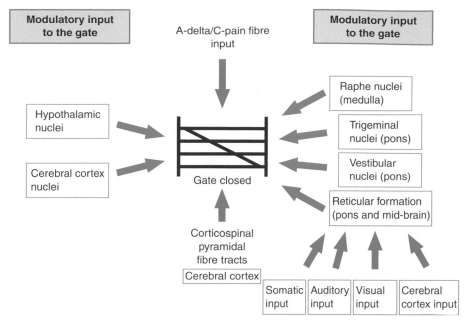

Figure 8.5 **Modulation of pain by descending fibres from higher centres**
The figure shows that the higher centre input to the gate dominates over the pain fibre
input so pain is not felt. However, this does not always operate

Q. Name the endogenous opioids mentioned in this chapter.

Biochemical and physiological subjectivity

Individuals have different capacities to produce various chemicals involved in the
transmission of pain. The person's genome is responsible for the production of
physiologically active enzymes necessary for the biochemical synthesis of pain-
producing substances, substance P, inhibitory endogenous opioids and inhibitory
neurotransmitters. If the genes responsible for the synthesis of pain-producing
substances or substance P were changed (i.e. mutated) or repressed, or the nociceptors become desensitized to pain-producing substances, then it would be possible to experience tissue injury without perceiving pain. Alternatively, people
may not report pain, despite tissue damage, if the genes necessary for the production of the endogenous opioids or inhibitory neurotransmitters are repeatedly
expressed, since high levels of them would close the gate. Conversely, high levels
of pain-producing substances (and consequently substance P) or low levels of
endogenous opioids and/or inhibitory neurotransmitters as a consequence of gene
activity or inactivity respectively would lead to pain hypersensitivity. Congenital
disorders of pain perception do exist; some people are born insensitive to pain,
whilst others feel pain without any detectable injury (Melzack and Wall 1996).

Sociopsychological subjectivity

Sociopsychological factors affect physiological processes and may be indirectly responsible for either opening or closing the gate. Social factors influence the development of the brain and these higher cortical centres may conceivably influence the physiological, neuronal and synaptic activity of the gate by influencing the descending control.

Anxiety is a state that may be genetically determined and/or environmentally socialized. In nursing literature it is well documented that elevated anxiety levels are associated with a patient's increased pain perception. The gate control theory would attribute this to depressed endogenous opioid levels, or to an increased substance P level; the former is most likely according to descending control theory.

Box 8.3   Application: care and anxiety

A patient's anxiety level is heightened with admission to hospital, the thought of the impending diagnostic procedures and, if applicable, surgery itself influences the individual's perception of pain (Hollinworth 1995). Perioperative care should aim to reduce the patient's anxiety levels before attempting to quantify the pain that the patient perceives. Perhaps, then, an appropriate action might be just to empathize, sit and support the patient in pain, since this physical assurance can have analgesic qualities.

Cultural differences in the perception of pain are also observed, and therefore need to be taken into consideration when assessing pain. This could suggest that past socializing experiences and individual conditioning have important influences on the subjective elements of pain. Socialization determines psychological behaviour, which could conceivably affect the output of endogenous opioids.

Box 8.4   Application: caring for all cultures

The practitioner should be concerned with management of a particular type of pain by using constant patient monitoring, rather than have different treatment regimens according to the patient's perception of their pain. The perioperative practitioner should be familiar with cultural differences when reducing the patient's anxiety prior to assessing the appropriate care to be implemented.

EXERCISES

1 Using a nursing dictionary look up the meaning of 'analgesia' and 'anaesthesia'.

2 Use Figure 8.4 to revise your understanding of the operational workings of the gate control theory of pain perception.

> **Box 8.5   Application: the process of hospitalization may even reduce pain!**
>
> The importance or meaning of a situation can affect one's perception of pain. Prior to entering hospital (particularly in an emergency) pre-admission pain can seem almost unbearable, whereas post-admission interviews indicate that the pain may have lessened or even disappeared. Perhaps the fear of a serious surgical operation results in a surge of endogenous opioid gene activity, resulting in high levels of these painkillers! If this is the case, then it demonstrates how environmental factors, such as the clinical setting, presence of doctors and healthcare professionals, and unfamiliar and possibly high technology equipment, may influence gene activity and subsequent opioid release, thus reducing or abolishing the pain.

The next section of this chapter reviews the site of action of analgesic agents and anaesthesia employed during perioperative care.

Perioperative pain management

The assessment and management of perioperative pain are critical skills for the surgical nurse; hence, the subjective nature of pain should be reflected in their approach to pain control. Unfortunately, many studies (e.g. Royal College of Surgeons and College of Anaesthetists Commission 1990; Field 1996) suggest that the nurse's knowledge of perioperative pain management is inadequate. However, as Carr (1997) reported, nurses are not the only group of healthcare professionals who demonstrate a lack of 'expertise' in providing analgesic relief. Carr reviewed the survey of twenty-seven medical schools by Marcer and Deighton in 1988, which revealed that four schools undertook no formal teaching on pain control, and the remainder averaged only 3.5 hours during a four-year course. The situation is improving (McCaffery and Ferrel 1997) but perioperative pain management remains a major problem!

Pharmacological pain management

The use of analgesic drugs is the mainstay of immediate perioperative pain management. The important aspects of pharmacological therapies are to provide the patient with sufficient pain relief to allow rest, relaxation, pain-free sleep, mobilization and to avoid the toxic effects of the drugs and the occurrence of breakthrough of pain (Torrance and Serginson 1997). The administration of regular, adequate doses will prevent the latter (see Figure 8.6a). If breakthrough pain occurs, the perioperative practitioner, while appreciating/considering the possibility of drug toxicity (see Figure 8.6b) may deem higher dosages necessary. Analgesic drug administration can be via a variety of routes: oral, sublingual, rectal, inhalation, intramuscular, intravenous, subcutaneous, transdermal, spinal and epidural. Intravenous drugs may also be administered using patient-controlled administration systems.

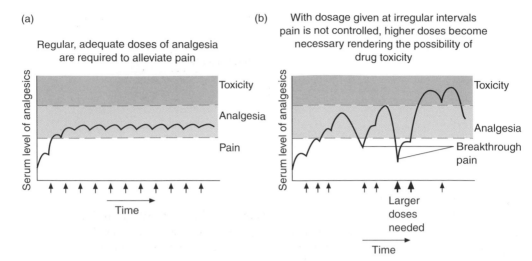

Figure 8.6 a **Drug administration in successful analgesia**
Note
Regular, adequate doses of analgesia are required to alleviate pain.

b **Drug administration in breakthrough pain**
Note
Analgesics given at irregular intervals may result in breakthrough pain. Higher doses may then be deemed necessary, rendering the possibility of drug toxicity.

Q. How is breakthrough pain prevented?

Perioperative pain may be managed using non-opioid and/or opioid analgesics. That is, if pain persists then the principles of the analgesic 'staircase' are employed in an attempt to improve pain control (see Figure 8.7). The choice of drug depends upon:

- the location, type and severity of pain experienced. In general, the non-opioid simple analgesics are administered to relieve mild to moderate pain; the non-steroidal anti-inflammatory drugs (NSAIDs) are used for generalized pains or local inflammation. Of the weak opioids, some are administered to relieve mild to moderate pain, others to relieve moderate to severe somatic pain, and the stronger opioids are used for severe somatic pain.
- its pharmacological mode and site of action.
- its potential toxic effects.
- the periods of perioperative care.

Non-opioids

Since NSAIDs do not have the side effects of opioid drugs (e.g. respiratory depression, inhibition of gastro-intestinal motility), they are useful alternatives in

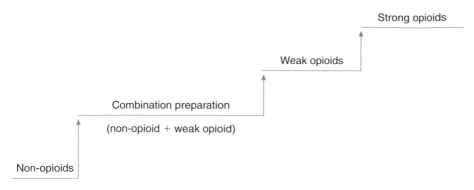

Figure 8.7 **The analgesic staircase**
The analgesic pathway may be used in order to reduce or abolish a patient's pain. That is, if the pain is not removed using non-opioids (e.g. paracetamol), then a combined preparation may be given (e.g. paracetamol + codeine phosphate). If the pain is still not removed, then weak opioids are given and if pain still persists, then a strong opioid is given

the management, for example, of postoperative pain, although they may be inadequate for the relief of severe pain. The non-opioids of particular frequent use in clinical pain management are paracetamol and the NSAIDs – diclofenac, ketoprofen, naproxen and ibuprofen (administered for mild to moderate pain relief) and ketorolac (administered for moderate to severe pain relief). Diclofenac is also used to *prevent* the occurrence of postoperative pain (Omoigui 1995).

Some non-opioids act outside the central nervous system in the periphery at the site of injury. For example:

■ paracetamol (or panadol) inhibits the formation of prostaglandins via inhibiting the enzyme prostaglandin synthetase (see Figure 8.8, i.e. Box A). Prostaglandins, if you recall, sensitize nociceptors (attached to the distal ends of pain fibres) to mechanical stimulation and enhance the effects of other pain-producing substances.
■ diclofenac and aspirin are thought to inhibit prostaglandin secretion from cells in the damaged area.
■ ibuprofen, ketoprofen, naproxen (also aspirin) provide analgesic relief via inhibiting the secretion of other chemical initiators (e.g. bradykinin, histamine) of pain (Omoigui 1995).

EXERCISES

List the pain-producing substances mentioned in the previous section.

Refer to a physiology textbook for a discussion of the lock and key theory of enzymatic action and competitive inhibition of enzyme activity.

Local anaesthetics

The preparation for patients who are undergoing regional anaesthesia is exactly the same as those who are having a general anaesthetic (see Chapter 7). Complications may arise during the perioperative period which may result in the patient needing a general anaesthetic.

Local anaesthetics provide regional anaesthesia by stabilizing afferent pain fibre membranes, via inhibiting the ionic fluxes required for the initiation and conduction of electrical impulses. In short, they cause a reversible block to conduction along the pain afferent nerve fibres (see Figure 8.8, i.e. Box C).

EXERCISE

Review your understanding of the activity/inactivity of the Na^+/K^+ ATPase pump during a resting membrane potential and an action potential respectively.

The local anaesthetics used vary widely in their potency, toxicity and length of effect, solubility, stability and ability to permeate mucous membranes. These variations determine their suitability for specific routes of administration, for example, infiltration, plexus, topical (surface) epidural or spinal block (Omoigui 1995).

EXERCISE

Use an anatomy and physiology textbook to identify the anatomy and physiology of the meninges, spinal nerves and vertebral column.

Spinal anaesthesia

Some patients will not be suitable for spinal anaesthesia, either because of the type of surgery being performed and/or pre-existing medical problems. Preparation of the patient is essential; a full explanation should be given because many patients may feel concerned about being awake during surgery or worried about the effects of the anaesthetic wearing off. Some patients have concerns about being anaesthetized and would prefer to be awake during surgery. Spinal anaesthesia is suitable for fit patients as well as those who are a high risk for a general anaesthetic.

EXERCISE

Consider the contraindications to spinal anaesthesia and suggest the reasons why spinal anaesthesia is inappropriate in each case.

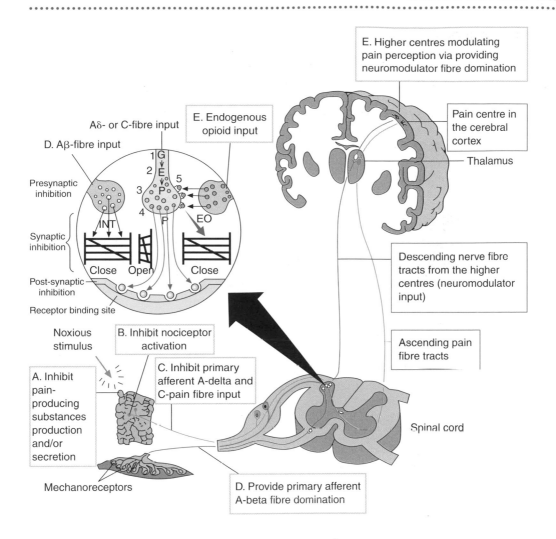

Figure 8.8 **Perioperative pain management: a gate control perspective**

Analgesia action is provided by:

1 *Inhibiting:*
   • the production and/or secretion of pain-producing substances (i.e. Box A),
   • nociceptor activation (i.e. Box B),
   • afferent pain fibre input (i.e. Box C).

2 *Replacing afferent pain fibre input domination via:*
   • promoting mechanoreceptors afferent fibre input (i.e. Box D), and/or
   • promoting neuromodulator descending fibre input domination (i.e. Box E).

The injection site for spinal anaesthesia can be at various levels of the lumbar (L) vertebra, a block at L2–3 will provide a suitable block for abdominal procedures, L3–4 block for the pelvis and legs. The local anaesthetic is injected into the subarachnoid space and mixes with the cerebrospinal fluid (CSF), which surrounds the surface of the brain and spinal cord. The CSF has a specific gravity much the same as water; if the local anaesthetic drug has a specific gravity much the same as CSF, it is known as an isobaric solution, if it has been made heavier than the CSF it becomes a hyperbaric or heavy solution. The specific gravity of the local anaesthetic and the patient's position are important factors in the spread and effect of the solution. The patient's physical and clinical condition, age, weight and height are used to determine the volume of the solution used. Pregnant women or patients who are in a poor physical condition may be given a lower volume of the solution.

For procedures that require a block that has a more localized action of a longer duration an isobaric solution may be used. Hyperbaric solutions will sink rapidly when injected into the subarachnoid space; if a high block is required the patient is placed onto their side for the injection, then turned onto their back following injection. This enables the hyperbaric solution to spread to the mid thoracic region; the solution is prevented from spreading further because the cervical end of the spine slopes upwards (see Figure 8.9). For a low block, the patient will be in the sitting position for the injection and remain there for a few minutes before lying down.

Bupivacaine is the most commonly used drug for spinal anaesthesia in the UK and is available in isobaric and hyperbaric solutions. Heavy bupivacaine has a specific gravity of 1013; it takes from ten to thirty minutes to take effect and lasts for two to three hours. It contains a solution of 0.5 per cent bupivacaine in 8 per cent glucose and is available in 4 ml ampoules.

Patients who have spinal anaesthesia may also be given sedation. Midazolam is often used. It provides an amnesic action (i.e. patients often remember nothing of their experience) and may produce respiratory depression, so close observation of respiratory function is necessary.

Complications of spinal anaesthesia relate to the spread of the drug within the CSF and include cardiovascular disturbances, respiratory depression, gastrointestinal disturbances such as nausea and vomiting, low urine output and hypothermia. The primary complication is profound hypotension. The most serious complication can be a total spinal respiratory paralysis and the patient will need to be intubated and ventilated. Later complications include headache, backache, urinary retention and, in rare cases, neurological disturbances.

Epidural anaesthesia

Epidural analgesia is commonly used during surgery, often combined with general anaesthesia to provide pain relief and aid muscle relaxation.

The local anaesthetic solution is injected into the epidural space blocking nerve roots in the epidural space at the site of injection. The effect is more localized than in spinal anaesthesia, providing a band of anaesthesia at the site of injection.

Spread T 10–S 5

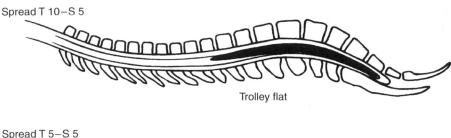

Trolley flat

Spread T 5–S 5

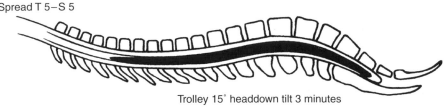

Trolley 15° headdown tilt 3 minutes

Injection – lying on side L3/4
Volume – 3 ml hyperbaric
Post-injection position – lying on back

Figure 8.9 **Effects of post-injection positioning on height of blockade**

The degree of anaesthesia is proportional to the volume of solution used; thus epidural anaesthesia requires a higher volume of solution than spinal anaesthesia to provide a therapeutic effect. It is of particular value for pain relief in obstetric care, post-operative pain relief, pain relief in other situations such as cancer pain and chronic pain conditions (British National Formulary 2002).

The local anaesthetics frequently used include bupivacaine, lignocaine chloroprocaine and procaine:

■ bupivacaine has a slow onset but will last for four to six hours, adrenaline may be added as it slows the absorption rate of the bupivacaine into the blood vessels producing a rapid onset and longer duration of action. Transmission is blocked at the nerve root and dorsal root ganglia. Bupivacaine is the principal drug for spinal anaesthesia in the UK (British National Formulary 2002).

■ lignocaine is the most widely used anaesthetic drug. It acts more rapidly and is more stable than other local anaesthetics. The duration of block (with adrenaline) is about one-and-a-half hours.

The primary side effect of an epidural is profound hypotension. Headache is a common side effect of epidural anaesthesia; leakage of the cerebrospinal fluid caused by dural puncture can cause severe headache within sixty minutes of puncture.

Box 8.6   Application: the role of the perioperative practitioner in epidural anaesthesia

Preparation for spinal and epidural anaesthesia must be the same as for general anaesthesia (see Chapter 7). Monitoring equipment for blood pressure, ECG and pulse oximetry must be available; drugs for general anaesthesia, intubating equipment, oxygen therapy and intravenous fluids should be prepared. Securing the IV access is a necessity and then the administration of a loading volume of 500–1000 ml crystalloid fluid prior to the commencement of spinal or epidural to combat potential hypotension. With the patient awake during surgery, all involved in the care of the patient should remember to modify their conversations. The patient must be accompanied at all times, never left alone as they may become anxious and agitated and require explanations and reassurance.

Opioid analgesics

Narcotics or weaker substitutes are classified as opioids because of their chemical resemblance to the body's endogenous neuromodulator opioids (i.e. the endorphins, enkephalins and dynorphins). Thus their analgesic site of action are the specialized opioid receptors located on the presynaptic membrane of the afferent pain fibres (see Figure 8.8, i.e. E pathway). Aspirin may also operate centrally on these opioid receptor sites inhibiting pain transmission.

Thomas (1996) stated that opioids provide analgesic relief by:

- depressing the appreciation of pain at the spinal cord level in the dorsal horn region, and/or
- stimulating activity in descending inhibitory pathways in the brain stem, and/or
- exerting mood-elevating effects, acting through the limbic system, and/or
- allaying anxiety.

Weak opioid analgesics

The weak opioid analgesics frequently used for the treatment of mild to moderate pain include codeine phosphate, co-dydramol, co-proxamol and co-codamol. These opioids are classified as narcotic agonists. That is, their analgesic site of action is at the endogenous opioid receptor binding sites.

Codeine phosphate is often used in combination with non-narcotic analgesics, such as paracetamol, for symptomatic treatment of mild to moderate pain. Twenty per cent of administered codeine is converted in the liver to morphine, which may account for its mild analgesic effects (Cass and Cass 1995): intramuscular (i.m.) administration of codeine has one-twelfth the potency of IV morphine.

Potent narcotic opioid analgesics

Potent opioid narcotics are the most effective analgesics and are particularly suitable for treating moderate to severe pain of somatic origin. Administration may be via intravenous, intramuscular, epidural or spinal routes. The advantages of epidural administration according to Omoigui (1995) are:

- lower dosages are needed,
- the effects are longer-lasting,
- mobilization is improved,
- the effects are limited to the immediate area, and
- respiratory depression resulting from the effects of the analgesics on the brain stem is minimized.

Narcotics produce other effects even in normal analgesic dosages. All narcotics produce powerful depression of the respiratory centres in the medulla oblongata and acute poisoning is always associated with slow, inadequate respiratory effort. Indeed it is this inhibition of ventilatory effort which endangers the life of these patients (naloxone is administered to reverse respiratory depression). All the drugs of this type are liable to induce nausea and vomiting because they have a stimulant action on the vomiting centre in the brain post-operatively, and this may necessitate giving anti-emetics (e.g. metochlopramide, cyclizine) at the same time as the opioids. Many of them produce characteristic stimulation of the parasympathetic nervous system, which results in constipation (British National Formulary 2002).

The analgesic qualities and side effects of opioids are a result of the opioid system being comprised of four distinct types of receptors: mu (μ), kappa (κ), delta (δ) and sigma (σ). Mu receptors are of two kinds – μ1 and μ2; the former are believed to mediate analgesia, whereas the latter mediate the side effects of respiratory depression, nausea, vomiting and constipation (Dobson 1997). According to Cass and Cass (1995) exogenous opioid stimulation of kappa receptors results in spinal analgesia, respiratory depression and sedation; stimulation of sigma receptors results in dysphoria, depression, hallucinations and vasomotor stimulation, but delta receptors are only stimulated by endogenous opioids. The opioids have different affinities for these receptors; for example, the affinity of morphine for the mu receptors is one hundred times greater than its affinity for the kappa receptors.

The dangers (particularly of respiratory depression) of the opioids have stimulated research into discovering analgesic compounds that minimize this side effect. A number of such compounds exist; for example, codeine phosphate and dihydrocodeine (DF118) are weak analgesics but are very good cough suppressants. They do however, cause constipation.

Opioid drugs may act as narcotic agonists (e.g. morphine, dimorphine), partial narcotic agonist (e.g. buprenorphine) and agonist-antagonist (e.g. nalbuphine) at any or all of the opioid receptors mentioned above (see Figure 8.8, i.e. pathway E). All of these drugs are used for the symptomatic treatment of acute severe pain, such as that caused by surgery. However, pethidine (an agonist-antagonist) is administered for the management of moderate to severe pain (Omoigui 1995).

EXERCISE

Reflect on your understanding of the terms 'agonist' and 'antagonist' used in this context.

The use of other narcotic agonists such a fentanyl is also very common. Fentanyl enhances the peripheral nerve block analgesic action of local anaesthetics, since this opioid drug also has weak local anaesthetic properties. That is, high doses suppress nerve conduction (via energizing the sodium/potassium ATPase pump) and have effects on opioid receptors in peripheral nerve terminals. Low dosages of fentanyl prevents pain via blocking nociceptor input and processing in the spinal cord.

Patient-controlled analgesia

Patient-controlled analgesia (PCA) forms an essential part of the healthcare professional's role in ensuring patient compliance. PCA allows patients to give themselves their own analgesia by activating a syringe pump. It provides a flexible form of pain control. The Royal College of Surgeons and College of Anaesthetists Commission (1990) acknowledged that the more the patient feels in control of their own pain management, the lower the requirement for analgesia. This is supported by Thomas *et al.* (1995) who claimed that PCA reduces pain dramatically post-operatively, and therefore promotes earlier discharge, hence the advocacy for PCA.

Thomas (1996) reported the following advantages of PCA:

- an apparent safe method of analgesic delivery,
- it bypasses the delays and deficiencies of the more conventional intramuscular injection method (Figure 8.10),
- it reduces anxiety; however, we would dispute this generalization, since not all patients feel comfortable being in control of their own pain relief.

The most frequently used route and drug for the control of acute post-operative pain, particularly following major surgery, is intravenous injection of morphine, although epidural and subcutaneous routes of administration are also used. The use of morphine is, however, dictated by the intensity of pain and therefore should be given when the weaker analgesics fail to provide relief. The use of diamorphine, pethidine and fentanyl is also very common. Other opioid analgesics either have a too long or too short duration of action for them to be utilized with PCA.

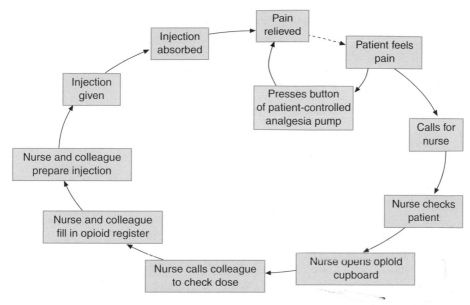

Figure 8.10 **The delays and deficiencies of the more conventional intramuscular injection method compared with the short circuit for patient-controlled analgesia**

Non-pharmacological techniques

Non-pharmacological techniques are more within the direct control of the health-care practitioner. They may be used in isolation or in combination with medically prescribed analgesics and are utilized as useful adjuncts to analgesia in the immediate post-operative period to reduce the side effects of drugs (Torrance and Serginson 1997).

A variety of non-pharmacological approaches to pain management exist. These include the provision of information and verbal support given to the patient, the therapies of touch, relaxation, distraction, imagery, biofeedback and transcutaneous nerve stimulation. While some of these are naturally the role of the nurse, others require specialized therapists. Of particular use in alleviating post-operative pain according to Torrance and Serginson (1997) are transcutaneous nerve stimulation, relaxation, distraction, massage and breathing techniques.

Non-pharmacological therapies provide analgesic relief by replacing the dominance of the afferent pain fibre to the pain gates needed to evoke a sensation of pain with:

■ inhibitory neurotransmitter domination (see Figure 8.8, pathway D), and/or
■ neuromodulator dominance (see Figure 8.8, pathway E).

The next section discusses these methods in more detail.

EXERCISE

The reader is advised to review Figures 8.3 and 8.5 from the previous section to gain maximum benefit from the following discussion.

Therapies that provide inhibitory neurotransmitter domination

Transcutaneous electrical nerve stimulation (TNS)

The technique in administering TNS requires very little training. It involves the electrical stimulation of the nervous system using a pulse generator, an amplifier and a system of electrodes (Figure 8.11). Although the mode of action of TNS is controversial, it has been generally claimed that:

■ the application of TNS stimulates the release of endogenous neuromodulator opioids,
■ it provides continuous analgesic relief by ensuring the domination of A-β afferent fibre input to the pain gates.

The place of this technique in today's management of post-operative pain is in great doubt. Its use has been abandoned by some health authorities, since it has been tried and found to be ineffective, thus emphasizing a subjective approach to the therapeutic management of pain (Clancy and McVicar 2002).

Touch

Touch therapies include massage, aromatherapy, acupressure or reflexology. On the whole, these therapies are regarded as being suitable for post-operative pain management (Torrance and Serginson 1997). Their analgesic qualities stem from encouraging domination of the A-beta afferents (with the mechanoreceptors at their distal ends) that input to the pain gates. It may even simply require holding a patient's hand, or lightly stroking the patient's forehead or forearm (Clancy and McVicar 2002).

Reflexology (i.e. the art of foot and hand massage) brings relief from stress while promoting the homeostatic reflexes associated with wound healing (see Chapter 4). Aromatherapy is the use of essential oils that have been extracted from plants to treat problems such as dyspepsia, nausea or flatulence, or they may be used as a relaxant (Torrance and Serginson 1997).

Touch therapies are designed to comfort and relax patients and thus enhance pain relief perhaps by enhancing the release of endogenous opioids. Touch promotes hypothalamic stimulation of the parasympathetic nervous system. Used correctly, touch can also relieve anxiety and reassure the patient that someone cares and understands (Torrance and Serginson 1997). One must be careful with this therapy, however, as the practitioner may invade the patient's 'personal space', and this may elevate anxiety levels. Thus, there is general support that the

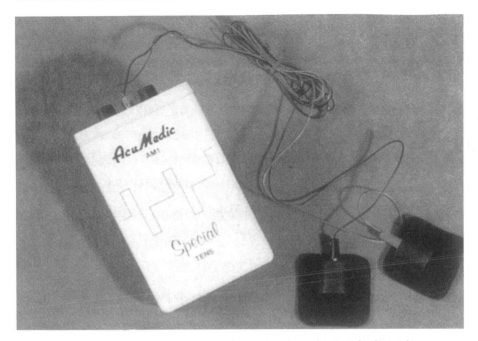

Figure 8.11 Transcutaneous Nerve Stimulation (TNS) machine with electrodes attached
Source: Photograph kindly supplied by the Acumedic Centre, London.

Q. Why is TNS not suitable for the control of all post-operative pain?

Q. How does the application of TNS machine relieve pain?

application of TNS and touch therapies provide dual analgesic relief through stimulating inhibitory neurotransmitter input and endogenous neuromodulator input to the pain gates (i.e. see Figure 8.8, D and E pathways).

Therapies that provide neuromodulator domination

The action of neuromodulators, e.g. endorphins, on descending fibre input to the pain gates form the psychophysiological basis of auditory and visual distraction and diversion therapies, hypnosis, biofeedback, counselling and placebo (Melzack and Wall, 1996).

Information giving and verbal support

Melzack and Wall (1996) stated that anxiety could produce a physiological response similar to acute pain. Thus, the criteria which should be part of any pain management plan is based upon establishing a good patient–nurse relationship so as to reduce the patient's anxiety and fears regarding:

- their impending stay in hospital,
- progression of their disease state,
- different pain relief techniques,
- potential complications.

The authors emphasize, however, that this information is to be provided in a manner that the patient can understand, to individualize care.

Anxiety promotes behavioural responses including muscle spasm and increased sympathetic activity. The former response compromises blood flow to tissues, causing ischaemia, thus increasing pain perception via the release of pain-producing substances, such as lactic acid (a by-product of anaerobic metabolism). The latter response can lead to pulmonary problems, increased cardiovascular work, altered muscle metabolism, increased oxygen consumption, and even death. Such behavioural responses can be minimized using the appropriate communication skills employed by the nurse to reduce patient anxiety and pain (Torrance and Serginson 1997). Perhaps, then, an appropriate nursing action might be just to empathize, sit and support the patient in pain since this physical assurance alone might have analgesic qualities (Clancy and McVicar 2002). Perhaps nursing care should aim to reduce the patient's anxiety levels before attempting to quantify the pain that the patient perceives.

The reassurance and communication skills used by nurses during a patient's stay in hospital probably enhances the neuromodulator descending fibre input to the pain gates.

Relaxation, distraction and imagery techniques

Relaxation is thought to remove or reduce pain by allaying anxiety. Relaxation and distraction techniques may act on both the higher centres involved in pain perception and the pain gating mechanism (see Figure 8.8). The Royal College of Surgeons and the College of Anaesthetists Commission (1990) acknowledged the value of relaxation in reducing post-operative pain and the consequential reduction in post-operative hospital stays.

Distraction draws attention away from the pain, focusing it to a pleasant sensory stimulus. The use of appropriate music can help the patient to relax and simple deep breathing exercises enhance this effect. It could be argued, however, that music must be pleasing to the patient to be beneficial; otherwise it may be a source of irritation, raising anxiety levels and thus the patient's perception of pain.

Imagery involves the patient focusing on a situation which is completely incompatible with pain. It may include one or a combination of all senses, incorporating a pleasurable sensation. This ranges from a simple sensation, such as getting the patient to describe a favourite pastime, to a complex mental visualization, which involves deep concentration on detailed tasks. Imagery promotes relaxation, which in turn alleviates or eliminates anxiety. The effectiveness of this therapy depends on the image used and the imagery ability of the individual patient concerned.

Table 8.1 The site of action of pharmacological and non-pharmacological analgesics during the perioperative period (Activity)

Therapeutic interventions	Site of action A	B	C	D	E	F	G
Non-opioid analgesics e.g. Paracetamol Diclofenac Aspirin Ibuprofen Naproxen							
Local anaesthetics e.g. Lignocaine Chloroprocaine Bupivacine Procaine							
Weak opiod analgesics e.g. Codeine phosphate Co-dyramol Co-proxamol Co-codamol							
Narcotic opioid analgesics e.g. Morphine Diamorphine Afentanil Fentanyl Pethidine							
Distraction and relaxation therapies							
Transcutaneous nerve stimulation							
Verbal support							
Imagery							
Touch therapies							

Notes: sites of action
A = Inhibition of prostaglandin synthetase
B = Inhibit prostaglandin sectretion
C = Inhibit bradykinins, histamine secretion
D = Activation of the 'sodium potassium ATPase pump'
E = Domination of the A-β fibre input to the pain gates
F = Blocking substance P's secretion
G = Domination of the descending neuromodulator fibre input to the pain gates

Q. Which letters are associated with the analgesic site of action of aspirin?

EXERCISE

Essentially successful pain management blocks the electrochemical impulses of the pain pathway at different locations en route to the brain's pain centre.

Using this information place a tick (✓) under the appropriate letter of Table 8.1 regarding the proposed operational activity of the following therapeutic interventions: Please note there may be *more than one* tick required for each intervention.

Summary

- In short, to perceive pain the afferent pain fibre input to the gate must dominate. Thus, to provide analgesic relief this domination must be removed via increasing the mechanoreceptors' afferent input and/or the descending neuron input to the gate.
- The concept of individualized pain relief is therefore based upon a knowledge of:
  - i the patient's background,
  - ii the progress of his/her illness,
  - iii the type and magnitude of the surgical procedure employed,
  - iv the area undergoing surgery,
  - v the durability/delicateness of the surrounding tissues.

  These are all relevant factors which need to be considered if perioperative pain management is to be successful.
- The aetiology and management of perioperative pain in patients is varied and sometimes complex. Management of pain, especially in the post-operative period, requires adequate pre-operative planning and skill on the part of the nurse in terms of both assessment and implementation of care.
- Therapies used fall into two categories: pharmacological and non-pharmacological.
- Analgesic drugs have actions that can be directly related to the neurophysiology of pain, especially in relation to the gating mechanisms put forward by Melzack and Wall in 1965.
- Non-pharmacological therapies have actions that remain debatable, though many can be related to the known neurophysiology. These 'alternative' or 'complementary' therapies provide potentially useful additional methods for pain relief, and can reduce the amount of analgesia used. The use of such methods recognizes that their psychosocial aspects can influence physiological processes and serve to highlight the subjective nature of pain. Therefore any approach employed is only effective if it is adapted to the patient's subjective needs (Clancy and McVicar 2002). If the patient is dissatisfied, then care must be reassessed and be adapted to ensure that the patient's comfort is achieved as soon as possible.

- The complexity of perioperative pain demands a multifaceted and multidisciplinary approach if the patient is to get effective pain relief. A prerequisite to good patient care is that the practitioner actually believes the patient. Unless this happens, one cannot get much further with pain assessment, and consequently its management.

- A good understanding of the individualistic nature of the patient's pain, underpinned by a sound knowledge of the neurophysiology of pain, is essential before practitioners attempt to plan and rationalize patient care.

- Biomedical and physiological research have provided significant understanding of some dimensions associated with pain, and psychological research has increased knowledge of the relationships between stress, anxiety and pain. Psychometric studies have generated various methods of measuring pain. However, because of the complexity of the phenomenon we label 'pain', there are many unanswered questions and continued research into the interrelations of these disciplines is the only way forward to unfold some of these mysteries.

Bibliography

Ackerman, C.J. and Turkiski, B. (2000) Using guided imagery to reduce pain and anxiety. *Home Healthcare Nurse* 18(8): 524–30.

Bell, F. (2000) A review of the literature on the attitudes of nurses to acute pain management. *Journal of Orthopaedic Nursing* 4(2): 64–70.

Bennett, G.J. (2000) Update on the neurophysiology of pain transmission and modulation: focus on the NMDA-receptor ... NMDA-receptor antagonists: evolving role in analgesia. Proceedings of a meeting sponsored by Algos Pharmaceutical Corporation, New York City. *Journal of Pain and Symptom Management* 19(1S Suppl): S2–6.

British National Formulary (2002) British Medical Association and the Royal Pharmaceutical Society of Great Britain. London. September.

Burden, N. (2000) *Ambulatory Surgical Nursing, Second Edition*. London: W.B. Saunders.

Carr, E. (1997) Overcoming barriers to effective pain control. *Professional Nurse* 12(6): 13–20.

Carrie, L.E.S., Simpson, P.J. and Popat, M.T. (1997) *Understanding Anaesthesia, Third Edition*. Oxford: Butterworth Heinemann.

Cass, N. and Cass, L. (1995) *Pharmacology for Anaesthetists*. London: Churchill Livingstone.

Clancy, J. and McVicar, A.J. (2002) *Physiology and Anatomy: A Homeostatic Approach, Second Edition*. London: Arnold.

Davies, J. and McVicar, A. (2000) Clinical practice. Issues in effective pain control 1: assessment and education. *International Journal of Palliative Nursing* 6(2): 58, 60–5.

Desjardins, P.J. (2000) Patient pain and anxiety: the medical and psychological challenges facing oral and maxillofacial surgery. *Journal of Oral and Maxillofacial Surgery* 58(10 Suppl 2): 1–3.

Dobson, F. (1997) Anatomy and physiology of pain. *Journal of Community Health Nursing* 2(6): 283–91.

Field, L. (1996) Are perioperative practitioners still underestimating patients' pain postoperatively? *British Journal of Nursing* 5(13): 778–84.

Fisher, S. (2000) Clinical feature article: postoperative pain management in paediatrics. *British Journal of Perioperative Nursing* 10(2): 80–4.

Gadsby, J.G. and Flowerdew, M.W. (2001) *Transcutaneous Electrical Nerve Stimulation and Acupuncture-like Transcutaneous Electrical Nerve Stimulation for Chronic Low Back Pain.* Oxford: The Cochrane Library.

Haker, E. (2000) A touch of pain. *Physiotherapy* 86(12): 618.

Hollinworth, H. (1995) No gain? *Nursing Times* 90(1): 24–7.

Horner, C. (1998) Acupuncture. *British Journal of Perioperative Nursing* 8(6): 33–5.

Jørgensen, H., Wetterslev, J., Møiniche, S. and Dahl, J.B. (2001) Epidural local anaesthetics versus opioid-based analgesic regimens on postoperative gastrointestinal paralysis, PONV and pain after abdominal surgery. Oxford: The Cochrane Library ,Issue 2.

Kittelberger, K.P. and Borsook, D. (1996) Neural basis of pain. Cited in Borsook, D., LeBel, A.A., McPeek, B. (eds) (1996) *The Massachusetts General Hospital Handbook of Pain Management.* Boston: Little, Brown and Company.

McCaffery, M. (1983) *Nursing the Patient in Pain.* London: Harper Row.

McCaffery, M. and Ferrel, B.R. (1997) Nurse's knowledge of pain assessment and management. How much more progress have we made? *Journal of Pain and Symptom Management* 14(3): 175–88.

McCaffrey, R.G. and Good, M. (2000) The lived experience of listening to music while recovering from surgery. *Journal of Holistic Nursing* 18(4): 378–90.

McQuillan, R., Finlay, I., Branch, C., Roberts, D. and Spencer, M. (1996) Improving analgesic prescribing in a general teaching hospital. *Journal of Pain and Symptom Management* 11(3): 172–80.

Mann, E. and Redwood, S. (2000) Clinical. Improving pain management: breaking down the invisible barrier. *British Journal of Nursing* 9(19): 2067–72.

Melzack, R. and Wall, P.D. (1996) *The Challenge of Pain.* London: Penguin.

Morton, N.S. (1997) *Assisting the Anaesthetist.* Oxford: Oxford University Press.

Omoigui, S. (1995) *The Pain Drugs Handbook.* London: Mosby.

O'Neill, O. (1998) Clinical feature article: the efficacy of oral analgesia for postoperative pain. *British Journal of Perioperative Nursing* 8(9): 5–8.

Parker, M.J., Urwin, S.C., Handoll, H.H.G. and Griffiths, R. (2001) *General Versus Spinal/Epidural Anaesthesia for Surgery for Hip Fractures in Adults.* Oxford: The Cochrane Library.

Parsons, G. (2000) Patient controlled analgesia was more effective than nurse controlled analgesia after cardiac surgery ... commentary on Gust, R., Pecher, S., Gust, A. *et al.* Effect of patient controlled analgesia on pulmonary complications after coronary artery bypass grafting. Critical Care Medicine. 27: 2218–23. *Evidence-Based Nursing* 3(2): 53.

Reilly, M.P. (2000) Clinical applications of acupuncture in anaesthesia practice. *CRNA – the Clinical Forum for Nurse Anaesthetists* 11(4): 173–9.

Rodgers, A., Walker, N., Schug, S., McKee, A., Kehlet, H., van Zundert A., Sage, D.,

Futter M. and Shepherd, S. (1999) Education focus: pain – developing an understanding and responding to it. *British Journal of Perioperative Nursing* 9(4): 157–63.

Royal College of Surgeons and College of Anaesthetists Commission (1990) *Report of the Working Party on Pain After Surgery*. London: RCS/RCA.

Stamford, J.A. (1995) Descending control of pain. *British Journal of Anaesthesia* 75(2): 18–26.

Stephenson, N.L. and Herman, J. (2000) Research brief. Pain measurement: a comparison using horizontal and vertical analogue scales. *Applied Nursing Research* 13(3): 157–8.

Szirony, G.M. (2000) A psychophysiological view of pain: mind–body interaction in the rehabilitation of injury and illness. *Work: a Journal of Prevention, Assessment and Rehabilitation* 15(1): 55–60.

Thomas, N. (1996) Patient controlled analgesia. *Nursing Standard* 10(47): 49–53.

Thomas, V.J., Heath, M.L., Rose, D. and Flory, P. (1995) Psychological characteristics and the effectiveness of patient controlled analgesia. *British Journal of Anaesthesia* 74: 271–6.

Torrance, C. and Serginson, E. (1997) *Pain*. London: Ballière Tindall.

Woolf, C.J. (1995) Somatic pain – pathogenesis and prevention. *British Journal of Anaesthesia* 75(2): 169–76.

Answer to multiple choice question

Q., p. 240

A	B	C	D
4	1	3	2

Index

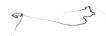